The International Library of Psychology

PSYCHOTHERAPY WITH CHILDREN

Founded by C. K. Ogden

First published in 1942 by
Routledge and Kegan Paul Ltd

Reprinted 1999, 2000, 2001 by
Routledge
2 Park Square, Milton Park, Abingdon, Oxfordshire OX14 4RN
711 Third Avenue, New York, NY 10017
First issued in paperback 2014
Transferred to Digital Printing 2006

Routledge is an imprint of the Taylor and Francis Group, an informa company

British Library Cataloguing in Publication Data
A CIP catalogue record for this book
is available from the British Library

Psychotherapy with Children
ISBN 13: 978-0-415-20919-9 (hbk)
ISBN 13: 978-1-138-00737-6 (pbk)

Abnormal and Clinical Psychology: 19 Volumes
ISBN 978-0-415-21123-9
The International Library of Psychology: 204 Volumes
ISBN 978-0-415-19132-6

CONTENTS

FOREWORD

CHILDREN WITH personality and behavior difficulties can be helped to help themselves. That is the theme of this book. I have not attempted to present a psychology of personality or an exhaustive discussion of comparative therapeutic methods. I am stating my point of view about therapy with children as that has grown out of the past seventeen years of clinical experience. What one has to say about therapy, like therapy itself, can never develop in isolation. Associated with me in the evolution of a therapeutic philosophy has been a staff of psychiatrists, psychologists, and social workers whose individual and combined contributions have been an integral part of the point of view contained in this book.

I have had several purposes in writing this book. Those clinics that have the opportunity to do careful therapeutic work with children and parents have a responsibility, I believe, to contribute to the meager literature on the nature and process of therapy. In drawing on the resources and material of the Philadelphia Child Guidance Clinic I have made available some of the experience that has evolved from our work.

More technical literature is needed for students who are taking training to enter active therapeutic work. The last two decades have seen a rapid expansion of child guidance clinics in this country. The staffing of these clinics with trained personnel is a large undertaking, and reliance has been placed on a few training centers in this country to meet material a point of view about the nature of childhood that will add to their sum of knowledge and understanding. I would like to emphasize, as I have already with pediatricians, social workers, and educators, that parents cannot, by the very nature of their relationship to their children, be therapists and try to function by imitating what therapists are in a position to do in their unique relationship to a child. Parents who attempt to be therapists introduce a confusion that follows when therapists attempt to fulfill the parent role with the children whom they treat.

Understanding the principles of therapy, and functioning in the role of therapist are two different things. Naturally the therapist has need of a theoretical basis if he is to become skillful in the discharge of his responsibilities. My interest in having more pediatricians, teachers, social workers, or even parents have greater understanding of the principles of therapy is to help them to be more effective in the job which normally is theirs to fulfill.

While my major emphasis in this book is on the participation of the child in the therapeutic process, it must be kept in mind that the value of what the child and therapist accomplish together is enhanced when the parent is an integral participant in the therapeutic procedure. We have learned not only how children can be helped directly, through therapy, but also how parents can be helped in their relationships with their children. This book deals with only one half of the therapeutic process in a child guidance clinic; the other half is still to be written by one skilled in the art of case work with parents.

Twenty years ago, when child guidance clinics were being established in various cities of the United States, under the sponsorship of the National Committee of Mental Hygiene and with the support of the Commonwealth Fund of New York, ways of helping parents and children were poorly defined. This was to be expected, since this was a new field of psychiatric endeavor. Psychiatry was beginning to be concerned not alone with mental sickness, but with the difficulties that spring up in the course of normal growth, particularly in children.

From the outset the child was the object of the studies and examinations carried on by psychiatrists, psychologists, and social case workers in order to determine the nature of his difficulty. In the earlier period of clinic development, however, change in the child was regarded principally as following upon changes in the attitudes of the parents, or upon modification of the external circumstances surrounding the child. This was the period when the primary emphasis focused on parents and what they did to shape the child's destiny. The behaviorists advanced the belief that a child with relatively normal equipment could be made into anything parents wanted him to be if they exercised their power, adequately and intelligently, in the first few years of the child's life. The child was seen as little more than a by-product of another's desire. With the ascendancy of this emphasis the parent was the center of educational and therapeutic procedures designed to make "bad" parents into "good" parents. This created a distortion of a parent's sense of responsibility since he was led to believe that the success or failure of the child rested entirely in his hands. Naturally this helped to inflate a parent's sense of importance when a child was a success, and precipitated in him abnormally guilty and deflated feelings when difficulties arose. The distortions at each extreme stemmed from the failure to appreciate the nature of growth and the participation of both child and parent in the child's development.

This false conception of the nature of childhood was reflected in the more authoritative and one-sided emphasis in the helping process. When a normal psychological growth was understood as a living process, that is, as "a differentiation of live people from each other," significant changes took place. No longer was the child just "brought up." Instead, he was regarded as an individual who could be helped to grow and to become a person in his own right. When therapeutic procedures took into consideration this principle, the child was included as an active participant in the relationship designed to help him. Instead of being seen as an object to be changed, he was accepted as a human being with the capacity to change.

The gradual incorporation of this different point of view about psychological growth into therapeutic procedures has brought about great transformations in the field of child psychiatry. This is particularly true when the therapeutic work with the child goes on concurrently with help given the parent to acquire a healthier relationship with the child. In this book I have tried to sum up my own experience, acquired largely in the Philadelphia Child Guidance Clinic. This organization functions as one unit in the important social and health resources available in the community. In the course of a year many hundreds of parents and children seek its services. They come from every section of the city and from every social and economic group. They are referred by other social and health agencies, by public and private schools, and by physicians. Large numbers of parents initiate this step themselves, and increasing numbers are referred by other parents who have used the services of the clinic.

In developing the most effective and skillful application of theory to the practical demands of the heavy case load in a community clinic, one important point must underlie all procedures. That is that procedures of working with parents and children retain their effectiveness only so long as they remain warmly human in their operation. The more skillful the therapist, the more natural and human he can be as he incorporates the theoretical background of his skill into the relationship with the child or parent.

Theory and practice in psychiatry sometimes have led a somewhat isolated existence and, when that happens, both suffer. Clinical practices provide the opportunity for the enrichment of theory which feeds back into service more understanding and refinement of method. In the material of this book, I have tried to maintain this close relation. Case material has been used freely in every chapter except in those at the beginning and at the end, and I have tried to weave together the practical and theoretical implications of the case illustrations. The first two chapters are devoted to a theoretical discussion of the nature of the normal psychological growth process, since the major theme of this point of view about therapy is that it is a specialized growth experience for a child and understandable through the same principles that apply to normal day-to-day growth.

Practically all the case material in this book has been drawn from the files of the Philadelphia Child Guidance Clinic. This organization has been an important training and research center in child psychiatry, and the staff has devoted a great deal of professional skill in building case records which bring out both the background facts about a parent and a child and the process whereby the helping relation unfolds. Without such records a book of this type would not have been possible. The facts in the cases used have been accurately drawn from the records and the only disguising has been in the names and identifying data.

References have been made to other contributions by students in this field and some parallels have been drawn between other ways of working to sharpen certain points I have wished to make. But I want to emphasize again that this book is not a study of all psychotherapeutic methods. It

wholes. In this process we see operating the principle of differentiation and the separating out of groups of cells with functional differences all related and interdependent. There is orderly purpose in this process. It is not simply cell division and reunion, a constant proliferation of cells without difference. This is the characteristic of cancer cell growth, where no cell differentiation occurs but only cell proliferation. The resultant mass has no function and becomes a foreign body. Normal growth, on the contrary, leads to the formation of functioning interrelated units which make possible an integrated whole that at birth takes the form of a living person capable of independent physiological existence.

In the original cell division a cell gives up a part of itself in order to go on growing. The principle of separation, as basic in growth and development, is manifest in that original biological phenomenon. The same principle of separation is operative in the birth process. Physiological differentiation and integration have proceeded to a point which allows the infant to function as a new living unity, and separation from the mother is necessary if the new functioning aggregate of cells which we call a baby is to go on living. Just as the original cell would die if it did not undergo division, so the infant would die if it were not divided from the mother. This is the end of one phase of growth with its more exclusive biological characteristics, and the beginning of a different phase that brings into operation new factors and new influences, and new functions emerge in both the infant and in the adults concerned with his birth.

Coghill has made important contributions to the study of the nature of biological behavior. Drawing his facts from animal experimentation, he observes that "the organism is first integrated as a total pattern without part-functions." Even early reflexes emerging as local reactions are under dominance of the total pattern and become partial or "individuated with a progressive restriction of the zone of stimulation to the amount needed for response." He states further that "inhibition first begins as a total reaction and dominates the whole organism." This gives way to local excitation and allows local or partial and appropriate reactions to take place. He concludes that "behavior develops in man, as it does in the amblystoma [salamander], by the expansion of a total pattern that is integrated as a whole from the beginning, and by individuation of partial patterns within the unitary whole." [1] Partial patterns of response, however, are made possible as the original whole gives up some of its original functions to a part as the new whole acquires its own different functions. This is not displacement of function but a basic phenomenon in cell differentiation with the growth and change of function as new cell aggregates reach the necessary stage of development.

In biological progression one can study the gradual emergence of these appropriate and partial functions of the parts of the larger whole from which they originate and for which they now work. The first reactions of the total organism thus made possible are significant. In keeping with Coghill's conclusions, it responds as a totality without the capacity, later acquired, for partial and more purposeful responses. When a young infant grasps for an object, the whole body is involved with the hand movement. In contrast is the later capacity to make fine and controlled move-

[1] Coghill, G. E., "The Early Development of Behavior in the Amblystoma and in Man," *Archives of Neurology and Psychiatry* (1929, v. 21), pp. 989–1009. "The Genetic Interrelation of Instinctive Behavior and Reflexes," *Psychological Review* (1930, v. 37), pp. 264–266. "Individuation Versus Integration in the Development of Behavior," *Journal of Genetic Psychology* (1930, v. 3), pp. 431–435. Quotations from the articles by Coghill are given in Evelyn Dewey's *Behavior Development in Infants: A Survey of the Literature on Pre-natal and Post-natal Activity* (New York, Columbia University Press, 1935), pp. 11–13.

ments with that hand. When a baby smiles he smiles all over; hand and foot movements are as noticeable as the play of facial muscles in this response. Biological differentiation proceeds from this integrated whole. Through this process, physical development brings about the ability to restrict movement to the particular parts needed for a response, allowing the others to proceed to the performance of their proper activities.

In this stage of the human growth process important breaking up and shifting of functions take place as the parts begin to assume their appropriate activity in their relation to each other. As the living individual emerges and begins to function as the integrated whole which is the new-born infant, he is brought into relation with his environment and becomes more than a biological entity. The term "psycho-biological" best describes this new phase of growth and living.

The moment an individual begins to live, unsupported by the physiological connection to the mother, new and significant influences and factors become operative. Consciousness of a separate self is awakened, and the infant gains a first awareness that while he is, in himself, an individual he is also closely associated with and related to others. This feeling is at first of an undifferentiated nature, in keeping with the status of infancy,[2] where the boundaries between what is self and not-self have not yet been clearly defined. With the opportunity to use his own muscles and do his own breathing and sucking and crying, the first steps are taken toward breaking up the totality of the infant's conception of self which is bound up in a larger whole, the mother.

[2] The Sutties speak of infancy as "a state of undifferentiated oneness with the mother. Its experience as far as it is continuous is an affective whole quite as well integrated in its way as its bodily organism."

Suttie, Ian D., "Mother: Agent or Object," *British Journal of Medical Psychology*, v. XII, no. II and III, 1932.

The infant is more than a physical unity influenced by reflex, chemical, and other physical stimuli. When he can respond as a separate biological integrate, he comes into relation with people and events, and is influenced by and in turn influences them. He becomes a social as well as a biological entity, capable of feeling. "Feeling," as I use it here to describe a quality in the infant, refers to an "organismic" [3] reaction that brings the individual into a state of awareness of his relationship with others. In its early manifestations, feeling is as undifferentiated as is the impression created by the use of the word. It is the sense of being alive, of being able to react to a stimulus with a pleasant or unpleasant overtone.

Mead speaks of feeling as "the lowest form of consciousness ascribed to a living thing." [4] What is implied is that when living forms enter into such a systematic process that they react purposingly, and as wholes to their own conditions, consciousness as feeling arises within life. Mead adds further: "Feeling is the term we use for this added element in life when the animal enters in some degree into its own environment." The infant does exactly this in the earliest reactions to stimuli. In responding as an integrated whole, the feeling of aliveness emerges in him. He and his environment no longer exist as a totality, one and indivisible. The first step in the final phase of differentiation between self and not-self emerges with this capacity to feel.

The capacity to have and to show feeling is a function taken over by the total organism. But its earliest expressions occur, of necessity, through the only medium available, the

[3] Child, Charles M., *Physiological Foundations of Behavior* (New York: Henry Holt & Co., 1924), p. 2, uses the term organismic to describe the behavior of the organism as a whole as distinguished from the behavior of single parts.

[4] Mead, George H., *Philosophy of the Present* (Chicago, Open Court Publishing Co., 1932), pp. 68 ff.

ture and nurture leads to a blind alley because of the attempt
to envision these great forces as having separate existence. A
clearer and broader conception of heredity and environment
will result when we cease trying to allocate to one or the
other the prime importance, and study them as inseparable
parts of one whole that acquires meaning and value in the
emerging self of a child.

This does not mean that these great forces cannot be
studied from one standpoint or the other. A child can be observed and studied in a laboratory, under controlled conditions such as Arnold Gesell of Yale has used so expertly.
Valuable data have been acquired by studying, in this way,
the orderly progression of functions in the growing child.
Equally valuable have been the studies of parental attitudes
and prejudices. Either set of data taken alone, however, fails
to give an adequate understanding of growth. The essential
dynamic has been obscured and the data lose their value
when an attempt is made to draw too sweeping conclusions.
The one tries to understand growth only as a biological
process. The other sees the child as a nonparticipating precipitate of the social forces playing upon him.

Further discussion of the interplay between outer and
inner forces in this differentiating process seems important
at this point. Emerging in the developing child is an awareness of a separate self, having a power which is his own but
which is experienced around the power and control of the
mother from whom the infant's self has emerged. The
vitalizing quality in the infant receives its first meaning and
direction through being experienced within this framework
of a living reality with others who can allow its different
value and, at the same time, guide and limit its expressions
in the child role. In this manner the child learns he does not
exist as a total force in himself. By the very nature of life

he feels his strength in relation to another person usually stronger and always different from him.

The concept of the super ego developed by the psychoanalytic school emphasizes that the outer—ideal-forming—force in the shape of parental morality and authority operates in a restrictive and inhibiting sense upon the primitive and unorganized instincts of the child. However, conceiving of the social forces as the outer, and the strictly biological (in the form of instincts) as the inner constitutes a cleavage that should be avoided if we are to understand what children are like. This procedure stresses the inherently bad in all that the child is originally, and postulates that only as the instincts are curbed and diverted from their theoretical goals and divested of their purpose can they become socially good and creative.[9]

From this point of view we would be led to believe that the ego or the consciously functioning self is the resultant, the sublimated precipitate in the battle that takes place between the primitive instinctive drives (id) and the restricting morality of external force in the form of parental prohibitions and cultural taboos. Rank, in setting forth his belief that the individual evolves his "ego ideal" from himself, states that "the ego is much more than a mere showplace for the standing conflict between two great forces," and concludes that the "ego is more than a helpless tool for which there remains no autonomous function."[10]

The view developed here concerning the nature of growth assumes that there is no such thing as "instinctive intuition."

[9] This point of view would gain support if we accepted Fenichel's statement that "parents remain as real persons in the real world but they are objects of aim-inhibited impulses only."
Fenichel, Otto, *Outline of Clinical Psychoanalysis* (New York, W. W. Norton, 1934), p. 412.
[10] Rank, Otto, *Truth and Reality* (New York: Knopf, 1936), p. 9.

is the emergence of a new and unique self, it is not in its normal manifestations an isolating process. In growth, separation and reunion go hand in hand, but the same analogy to the original cell division still holds. Human growth is a slow process, occurring in the supporting framework of one relation with another. The slower period of development, characteristic of man, reaches its peak in more highly organized cultures. The period of infancy and dependence is longer, and from that fact arise the greater strength and versatility of modern man.[16] Children are not thrust into responsibility too early nor forced to be adults before their time. But there is another aspect also, centering about the greater difficulties a modern child has in "giving up" his infancy. The source of greater strength which a slower period of development allows can also be a source of weakness for the child since there are more opportunities and temptations to prolong the period of dependence beyond the period of needing it.

Infancy is not merely a "flag station" on the road to a more mature period, to be passed by as quickly as possible. The infant who has gained real satisfactions in this period, through the love and direction of parents, will be one who can move away from it with the least turmoil. The fear inherent in accepting the new and untried and leaving the old and familiar is balanced, in the normally developing child, by the growth-inducing satisfactions gained from the old which he can now give up. The infant who has been given

---

of the Oedipus Complex: "Wherever that complex is found to occur it owes its origin to cultural factors." p. 388.

[16] Briffault called our attention to this when he said, "It would appear that the congenital superiority of what are regarded as the higher races of man consists essentially in a slower rate of development, owing to which the fixative force of natural heredity is counteracted by a more prolonged, modifying operation of the social environment."
Briffault, Robert, *The Mothers* (New York, Macmillan, 1931), p. 35.

a real chance to be an infant will be a healthier child emotionally.

The temptation and desire of some parents to exploit and overstimulate unusual abilities cause some children to be rushed through infancy too rapidly. This is apparent in the pride of the father and mother who tell of a child who never used "baby talk" but articulated words with clarity from an early period, or who brag about a child who was trained to bladder control before the first few months were over. These are samples of achievements of dubious value, as they are not natural for the level of development at which the child was. Too frequently such a child will begin to talk "baby talk" or develop enuresis when he is four or five years old, much to the dismay of the parents who had come to regard their child as "grown up." An unhappy, neurotic girl of fourteen formulated her major complaint as being that she was "born too soon," and it was true that she never had had the chance to be an infant which fact, in turn, distorted the satisfactions of being a child.

Trying to recapture an earlier period of development at a later period is a common human desire, and it serves to reemphasize, by contrast, the growth-inducing values that emerge as individuals can be helped to function in roles appropriate for each phase of development. The family structure provides the most natural setting in which this occurs, and attention can now be directed to the dynamic influence of family life in determining the function of the father-mother-child-roles, the three basic roles in every culture.

2

THE FUNCTION OF THE FAMILY
IN THE CHILD'S GROWTH

DEFINITIONS OF human relationships[1] occur only in the living experiences of individuals functioning in roles appropriate to their biological grouping (sex, age) and to social adequacy acquired by growth and training. Around the clarifications of these functional and biological differences for each human being occur the most significant events of individual and group living. The comparisons, imitations, rivalries, satisfactions, and disappointments constitute the drama of humans living together and finding the means to maintain their individual status in a world of others. The interrelation between the big and the little, the young and the old, the male and female invests these universal descriptions of difference with dynamic significance for every human being. The child in adapting to these evidences of difference defines and gives meaning to his own individual role which he lives in relationships with others. In the process of defining this role each individual, whether child or adult, becomes an integral influence in defining the roles of others who complete his social setting. (In Chapter X I have used

[1] Part of the following material was given by the author as a separate paper at the annual meeting of the American Orthopsychiatric Association in New York, February, 1941, and published in the *Journal of Orthopsychiatry* (January, 1942) under the title "Dynamics of Roles as Determined in the Structure of the Family."

a passage from Thomas Mann's *Joseph in Egypt* to illuminate this point.)

Malinowski emphasizes "the impossibility of envisaging any form of social organization without the family structure." [2] This is the indispensable unit of all social organization throughout the history of man. The family gains this dynamic significance for human nature because, in its functioning, a setting is provided for the definition and conservation of human difference and is given objective form in the different but related roles of father-mother-child, the basic roles in any culture. Biological factors provide the framework in which an individual functions in a role, but cultural influences in the form of law, taboos, rituals, and custom— the precipitates of human experience—give direction and meaning to the emerging self. The universal interplay between the biological and cultural forces gives the individual a sense of his own uniqueness. Thus man becomes not merely a recapitulation of the past, but creator of a new force that gives meaning and form to the ever new in life.

The conception and birth of a child bring, inevitably, a realignment of sentiments of the two adult members of the group. Their roles as husband and wife assume different direction and significance in the new status of father and mother. The arrival of the child throws into sharper relief functional differences, and these new functions focalize certain psychological tensions, well portrayed in the original Oedipus myth used so extensively as an analogy for the family drama. The recurrent repetition of this drama throughout the history of man provides both opportunity and necessity for parents to develop their adequacy to function in their adult roles, giving direction to the growth steps of their progeny as they gradually achieve their own maturity in

---

[2] Malinowski, Bronislaw, "Kinship," *Encyclopedia Britannica*, v. XIII, p. 403 (14th edition).

roles appropriate to their changing status. The functioning of the family unit toward the achievement of this basic goal has not been left to chance and individual responsibility, but has been defined by laws, customs, and taboos which, although general in nature, always apply to a particular mother and father and their children. These definitions shift and change and, in some respects, vary radically in different cultures. But they always provide social support to the roles in which individuals find, through their own experience, their way of living.

Benedict points out that "no individual can arrive even at the threshold of his potentialities without a culture in which he participates." [3] One of the important differences, however, between primitive and modern culture revolves around the social definition of this participation. In primitive cultures, roles have a more fixed status. Rituals and customs prescribe more clearly the functioning of the parents in their respective roles. The carrying out of these social sanctions gives them the status that the parent in our culture usually acquires with greater self-consciousness and purpose. The modern parent has more freedom to define his own way of living the role. Consequently he gains a different feeling of responsibility and of individual ownership of what is achieved. One example may clarify this distinction. The couvade,[4] which has had different forms among primitives, when it was carried out by a father gave him a status in primitive groups. In the usual form the father took to his bed and was waited on while the mother was giving birth to the child. The important thing to be considered here in the couvade is that the father acquires a status, not through functions normally belonging to the male role, but through

---

[3] Benedict, Ruth, *Patterns of Culture* (Boston, Houghton-Mifflin Co., 1934), p. 253.

[4] For more complete discussion of the couvade *see* Crawley and Besterman, *op. cit.*, II, pp. 177–88.

this ritualistic denial of difference by imitating, in this ceremony, the role of the mother at childbirth. Thus he acquired significance for his own contribution in the birth process.

This shift in the relative importance of cultural and individual determinants of roles, of which there is ample evidence in successive generations in our own country, has led to greater individual creativeness, but through it also has come about more of the turmoil observed by the psychiatrist in clinical work where a father, mother, and child have difficulty in carrying out their individual but related roles. This change in emphasis serves to throw into sharper relief the obvious fact that human roles always are defined and are given meaning through the inseparable relation that exists between the cultural supports and the individual who, in adapting, gains in himself, through his own experience, a sense of his own difference. These influences vary only in degree and can never exist as separate forces.

Another fact of significance is that one definition of difference in these roles has developed throughout cultural history without essential modification. This is the incest taboo.[5] Why this rule should maintain its universal place in defining human relations, particularly in family life, has been the subject of considerable discussion and disagreement, and many theories have been advanced to explain it.[6] A clearer explanation of this firmly established proscription throughout mankind seems to emerge with a functional understanding of the difference in roles. The conventions, laws, and taboos existent in every social group do not determine human differences. Instead they define and protect them, since

[5] Freud devotes the entire first chapter of *Totem and Taboo* to tracing this development. Vide *Basic Writings of Sigmund Freud* (translated and edited by A. A. Brill, New York, Modern Library, 1938), pp. 807–20.

[6] The various theories advanced to explain the incest prohibition are discussed by J. C. Flugel, *The Psychoanalytic Study of the Family* (London, Hogarth Press, 1929), ch. XVII.

the virility of any culture stems from the inalterable fact of human difference. Man and woman, adult and child, perceive value and meaning in their difference through living together in roles consistent with their biological status.

The incest rule, particularly as it applies to intrafamily relations, has emerged from essential biological differences which, in turn, determine important functional differences in the roles of father, mother, and child. The family is and has been the social institution in which these roles are defined by the living experiences the individuals have together. Tozzer has pointed out that "the family stands apart as the one human institution where physical functions and psychological ones as well clearly define the status of the two main members." [7] When the adults have found worth in their own different but related roles, they provide the medium in which the child can find, in his own growing, the values of being a child. Malinowski, who has made so many important contributions to functional anthropology, states that "incest is incompatible with the establishment of the first foundation of culture. In any type of civilization in which custom, morals and law would allow incest, the family could not continue to exist." [8]

Why is this true? It is not because of biological contraindications to incest, since most anthropologists agree in questioning the deleterious effect of in-breeding and point out that it is common in animal life. Nor can this truth be explained on the theoretical basis of a universal incestuous attachment of the child to the mother, the repression of which leads to this universal law. The incest prohibition is both the recognition and the protection of essential differences

---

[7] Tozzer, Albert, *Social Origins and Social Continuities* (New York, Macmillan, 1925), p. 92.

[8] Malinowski, Bronislaw, *Sex and Repression in Savage Society* (New York, Harcourt Brace, 1927), p. 251.

in emotionally related roles. The family can function only through the individual differences of its members, determined and experienced in the three basically related roles of father, mother, and child. When these differences are denied or obliterated, even by one member of the group, the configuration essential for normal living changes, and confusion and chaos result. This happens not only when the incest barrier is removed, but, just as clearly although with subtler effects, when individuals fail to find value and satisfaction in being what they are, and attempt to deny their own difference by assuming the role of another.[9]

In everyday life and particularly in clinical work, we see the confusion that ensues when the mother, dissatisfied with and fearful of her femininity, attempts to be the father and the man; when the father, uncertain of his ability to attain masculine status, exaggerates or denies the functions of the father role; when the child, in discovering his difference, attempts to deny it, and to cling to the mother or father as an undifferentiated part of himself; or when both parents have too great zeal to give a child "freedom" on the theory that repression is bad. In each of these situations there is failure to provide the child with the essential support and direction he requires and receives from a father and mother functioning normally in their own roles. In these dramas of living are provided clinical evidence for the conclusions reached by many anthropologists that the incest barriers or other functional definitions rooted in essential human biological differences are culturally determined. The incest barrier has nothing to do with the creation of these functional differences; it is evidence of these differences, and of how cultures define and protect them.

[9] This point was discussed in the author's paper on "Homosexuality in Relation to the Problem of Human Difference." *American Journal of Orthopsychiatry*, v. X, no. 1 (January, 1940), p. 129-35.

The Oedipus analogy, first used by Freud [10] in 1899 and since occurring extensively in psychoanalytic literature to explain the nature of the family, takes on wider and more significant meaning when it is seen as the drama of individuation and self-differentiation rather than as the solution of a theoretical instinctive incestuous attachment of the growing child to the mother. [11] A broader and more positive understanding of growth follows from a functional conception of the interrelated and concurrently operating forces in mother and father and child as they live their appropriate roles together. In the failure of one or more roles, the entire balance of the family is disturbed.

The commonly accepted version of the Greek myth provides a clue to this broader concept. The sequence of events in the myth was initiated by the parents, not by the child. The father, [12] told by the oracle (his own fear) that an unborn son would grow to be his murderer and marry his wife, wanted this potential danger removed at birth and given away to the shepherd. The father's fear had nothing to do with the eventual marrying of the mother by the son, but

[10] Freud, Sigmund, *Interpretation of Dreams*, as reprinted in *Basic Writings of Freud* (Modern Library, 1938).

[11] This latter focus on the instinctive organization of the child, with the parents in the roles of inhibitors and objects of purposes "most foul, unnatural," (Sophocles, "Oedipus Rex") presumes an instinctive function which the infant does not possess. To the role of father and mother in this interpretation of the Oedipus drama are assigned mainly negative and repressive values. Reference has been made (p. 25) to the emphasis Fenichel placed on parents as "objects of aim-inhibited impulses only." This is consistent with the psychoanalytic use of the Oedipus analogy which stresses the repression, by the child, of the objectionable instinctive impulse which would lead, unless sublimated, to an incestuous attachment to the mother. This emphasis stresses that growth can proceed only as the parents are "desexualized." This distortion occurs when we view growth as an inner unfolding of instinctive drives unrelated to their function.

[12] In some versions it is the father who gives the child to the shepherd. In another version the mother gives the child away upon seeing how sorely distressed Laius had become. In both versions it is the father's distress and fear that are important.

sprang from a fear of losing himself in the new father role in which he would have to function following the birth of a boy child. He faced the need to prove his adequacy, a need recurring in each life cycle as a man and a woman function in the role of father and mother to their children. Parents' uncertainties and emotional entanglements, focused and intensified around the child, throw out of balance the necessary functions of mother and father roles. The reactions of the child to these disturbances can distort further the family drama and lead, in some instances, to the determined, possessive drives frequently misinterpreted as incestuous in origin, but which actually may and do take on this meaning through the development of the struggle itself.

Ample illustration of the operation of these influences in modern family life can be drawn from the records of any child guidance clinic. We see how mothers strive to hold children as undifferentiated parts of themselves and thus fail to give the natural love and direction children need to guide them in the affirmation and achievement of their own differences. We observe how a child may struggle against the demands of growth and attempt to retain the mother as a symbol of infancy, resenting strongly the father with whom he must share the mother. These are common clinical problems. Yet these reactions of father, mother, and child cannot be studied and treated as separate phenomena since they cannot, by the nature of life, be separate. They are aspects of the drama of growth and of self-definition, not the outcome of a hypothetical incestuous attachment of the child to the mother. It cannot be, if we accept the belief that instinct has meaning only in terms of its function.

In sexual activities and in other ways the child becomes aware of his functional and individual differences from the parents. He may fight against the acceptance of this difference, and may even carry the struggle to the point of trying

framework which continues to define the world to which he is so closely related and the place he can begin to take in it.

Limitations or bounds have, basically, positive value. They provide a foundation for growth not because they restrict instinct expression, but because they give *meaning* to such expression, and allow for creative and purposeful use of emergent capacities and powers. It is true that the child, in varying degree, may try to retain in the mother the outgrown symbol of his infancy, and that the mother may find satisfaction in retaining that relationship. But in the normal process of growth, in which some struggle is inevitable, the child gains awareness of his own separate being and finds that he can use this power assertively, but he finds also that he can yield without surrendering his strength altogether and becoming the passive product of another's desire.[15]

This struggle in the parent and child relationship can become the intense one seen commonly in clinical practice. The child may fight against giving up his infantile relationship to the mother, fearing the separateness of living, and finding his fear a most effective weapon with which to maintain the old position, to preserve the completeness of the identification which early infancy allows and requires. He fights against giving up the mother as a symbol of his own undifferentiated self. Putting it another way, the child's effort is directed against the acceptance of his own self as having a separate identity, which implies a creative use of

[15] Robinson has given us a clear formulation of the positive aspects of identification in this statement: "Enlargement and enrichment of the self can be seen as the result of the process of identification as the individual takes into his own psychological structure aspects of the different wholes of which he has become a part. As the self becomes organized through separation and deprivation experiences it gains greater awareness of its own wants as inside and the objects which satisfy, oppose, deny or punish as outside." Robinson, Virginia P., *Supervision in Social Case Work* (Chapel Hill, University of North Carolina Press), p. 19.

his own difference. The guilt activated in this struggle centers around this fact of being different, acceptance of which would mean giving up the projection of self in the object with which he is too completely identified.

In most behavior problems in children this represents the ascendancy of a negative factor in the identification of child with mother and mother with child and is distortion of a basically positive and universal process. It is the positive affirmation of self—with the mother as object of identification and her acceptance of herself as a part of the child's early reality—that enables the child both to satisfy his need for dependence yet to develop toward the independence which human growth implies. The mother can define her own separateness by allowing the child not only to discover that the source of these needs lies in himself but that he is able to use his own capacities to satisfy them. This can be illustrated in the daily experience of any normal mother. The child learns to use the current language form because of a need to give more articulate indication of what he wants. If the mother feels the need to anticipate the child's wants and does not let him have the preliminary discomfort of making known what he wants, the child has less need for language and may actually postpone speaking for many months.

A child moving toward a more real feeling and acceptance of himself finds many ways of reinforcing his emerging and not yet adequate capacity to deal with his own realities. I have already mentioned the need of a child to affirm his emerging self in others, usually members of the family. Thus he can feel, with more safety, the increasing awareness of his own separateness and difference from those with whom he has necessarily been identified and whose support has provided the framework for growth.

The growing child has other sources of support which he

finds useful. There is a feeling of oneness between a child and his possessions. In exaggerating their power and bigness he enhances his own uncertain feeling of adequacy. He may draw a picture of a snake or a giant, and feel the power of the object as his own. Here again we observe interesting parallels between child and primitive man, who is able to reinforce his own powers through investing elements in his environment with the opposite of the lacks he perceives in himself. When going into battle, some primitives sprinkle their bodies with holy water, and certain tribes eat snakes to acquire bravery. The people of Surinam wear iron,[16] the strong substance, and thus acquire its strength. These objects and the individual merge, for the primitive, into an indivisible whole, as he possesses the power of the object as his own. While the growing child holds a more clearly defined distinction between the real and the unreal, he can nevertheless draw from the unreal a reinforcement needed for growth.

A concept of growth which sees it as a living, dynamic, functioning process seems essential if we are to give balanced consideration to the facts in both the biological and psychological areas. Growth cannot be viewed merely as a biological process because of the very nature of the totality which characterizes the early reality of the child. But it is a biological process occurring within a framework of relationships and events which gives meaning and direction to the emerging self of the child. This emerging self is not a pawn moved around by external influences designed to restrict the primal instinctive forces; in that point of view there is little place for the real and spontaneous values of the self. These outer and inner forces are, instead, a totality, and the child acquires through their operation a feeling of what

[16] Crawley, Ernest, and Besterman, Theodore, *op. cit.*, p. 150.

belongs to self and what belongs to the outer world in which
he experiences his capacities. The dynamic that lies in the
differentiating nature of growth is lost sight of when the
outer (parental authority) is viewed only as restrictive
means of blocking instinct expressions. This emphasis assumes that all instincts in the human are bad and must
have their basic character and purpose changed before an
individual can establish a friendly and socially acceptable
place in a world of other persons. This leads to the blind
alley of viewing growth as an avoidance phenomenon, and
all training and education as the subjugation of the "little
savage" that the infant is regarded as being.

Instincts undergo change as appropriate functions emerge
under the directing influence of a particular culture and
particular parents. This does not mean that change is motivated only by what is prohibited. The resistance to change,
as a means of perpetuating infancy or of growing only in
one's own terms, as it were, may invest change with all the
negative, aggressive elements encountered clinically, and
may even develop the classical Oedipus situation between
child and parents. That is what the growth process may become, under certain circumstances, not what it customarily
is. I hold with Meyer, who sums up the more positive view
this way: "The philosopher who thinks that man will not
act unless prompted by pain and conflict maligns nature as
does he who trusts only an arbitrarily hypothesized unconscious. We have a right to speak of a wider and perfectly
natural uncomplicated spontaneity, just as we have a right
to speak of natural growth as a differentiation of live individuals." [17]

The self, then, can be viewed not merely as a precipitate,

[17] Meyer, Adolf, "Spontaneity," *Proceedings Illinois Conference Public
Welfare*, Mental Hygiene Division, 1933, p. 25.

This book emphasizes the values of what people have and how they can be helped to use their present capacities to effect their own changes. We begin with the fundamental thesis that no one can effect change in another person without the participation of the person in whom change is desired. This is as true of children as it is of adults. The focus lies in what people can be helped to achieve and not in what is done to, or for, them to bring about change. Taft [2] has this clearly in mind when she states: "The word therapy is used instead of treatment because in its derivation there is not so much implication of manipulation of one person by another." Therapy is concerned with a process and must give full recognition to the essential participation of the patient in this process. As Taft says: "Therapy cannot do anything to anybody—hence can better represent a process going on, observed perhaps, understood perhaps, assisted perhaps, but not applied."

It is simple to tell people in distress what is wrong and what should be done to correct their mistakes, yet usually it is as ineffective as it is simple. Parents and children reveal rather quickly the sources of their difficulties, and trained people readily see what has been wrong. But there is no therapy in that understanding per se, essential as it is for the orientation of the therapist. It is what the patient can begin to do in the clarifying and understanding medium of a relationship with the therapist that must be the focal point of interest, if the therapist is to avoid the pitfalls awaiting the "synthetizer," or the authoritarian who knows the answers and cajoles the patient into accepting them.

A short example drawn from the adult field will illustrate this. A woman in early middle life became disturbed when the offer of a new position forced upon her an awareness of being deeply involved in a relationship with another woman.

[2] Taft, Jessie, *Dynamics of Therapy* (New York, Macmillan, 1933), p. 1.

Faced with the necessity of choosing between the job, which would take her to a distant city, and the other woman, she sought help. She was told that she must break up the relation, move away and broaden her base of living by having more friends, if she really desired a healthier life. Theoretically, the advice may have been sound enough but the patient had no part in building the new plan. She was told what to do. As a result she was more disturbed. With a different therapist the question as to what she should do arose with greater urgency. She was helped to work on what she herself was able and ready to do. The actual making of the decision was a secondary matter. The result of this change in emphasis was a clearer, recaptured feeling of her own integrity through which she arrived at a plan that was her own. Out of her disturbance and the seeking of help, she gained a clearer definition of herself. In arriving at her own plan of action she not only solved the pressing job question but also regained possession of herself. The first approach was based on an urge to do something in order to bring about change. The second, stemming from and illuminating the fundamental thesis of this book, permits the change to emerge from what the individual can be helped to do. Here the therapist was in a position to invest with positive meaning the fact that the woman was disturbed and that she took the initiative in seeking help. Therapy begins when the therapist is brought into a relationship as a supporting and clarifying influence around the patient's need and desire to gain or regain a sense of his own worth.

Among the phrases that have crept into modern psychological language is the term "relationship therapy." In a sense this is misleading because it seems to imply a special brand of psychological therapy. All therapy involves a relationship between patient and therapist. The differences in theory and practice arise around the values and uses that are assigned to this relationship. Throughout the history of psychotherapy, different uses have been made of the doctor's relation to a patient. I shall refer but briefly to two of these by way of contrast rather than in an exhaustive discussion of their values and limitations. It is the third which represents the major emphasis in this book.

The therapeutic relationship can be used authoritatively. This use is evident in the more direct efforts to tell a patient what to do, to lay out plans for his recovery and to fit him to a regime designed to ameliorate his difficulties. In less direct forms we see it in the subtle use of suggestion, in hypnosis or in the application of formulas and beliefs, such as "a military school will help" or in slogans such as "don't worry" or "be calm." The authoritative use of a relationship is characterized by the frank and purposeful utilization of an opportunity to bring about change. In this sense therapy has more in common with those methods which depend upon the employment of an external force, like a drug, to induce changes in behavior.

The second use of the relationship, which might be termed the "genetic" or "causal," strives to utilize the therapeutic experience as a means of getting at the historical background of the difficulties, of making conscious the unconscious trends and drives and re-creating the past in the therapeutic situation in order to release anxiety bound up with these earlier experiences. The emphasis is on the establishment of the "transference," from which insight proceeds. The focus is directed toward what the patient *was* in order to help him clear up conflicts in his present self. "It endeavors to bring unconscious conflicts to consciousness and aid in their resolution by placing them under the governance of the ego." [8]

The third use will, as I have said, receive the major em-

[8] Pearson, G. H. J., and English, O. S., *Common Neuroses in Adults and Children* (W. W. Norton, 1937), p. 185.

phasis in this book, and the rest of this chapter attempts to clarify its clinical application and the theory underlying it. Here the therapeutic relationship is conceived as an immediate experience. The therapist begins where the patient is and seeks to help him to draw on his own capacities toward a more creative acceptance and use of the self he has. While maintaining an interest in understanding what has been wrong, the therapeutic focus is on what the individual can begin to do about what was, and, more important, still is wrong. Therapy emerges, then, from an experience in living, not in isolation but within a relationship with another from whom the patient can eventually differentiate himself as he comes to perceive and accept his own self as separate and distinct.

This point of view is rooted in a philosophy of responsibility, a belief that people have within themselves, irrespective of what has gone before, capacities which can be utilized creatively to effect harmonious relations with the realities of their living. These qualities are tested in the therapeutic process. The very assumption or expectation that the patient take a part in bringing about change sets in motion responses from which changes can emerge. How does this come about? In this unparalleled situation, therapist and patient are brought into a significant relation with each other. The therapist has assigned to him, by the very nature of his role, the power to effect change. The patient, by virtue of his difficulty and his admission of a need to change, places himself in the position of *being* changed. In fact, he frequently comes expecting to be changed by the "expert's" skill. The reactions stirred in the patient, when he finds himself in a situation that both allows and expects him to be an active participant in his own changing, are both varied and significant. One patient dodges all responsibility and leaves everything to the therapist when he says, in effect,

out external prompting or coercion is what interests us above everything else." [7] This places the patient in the center of an experience designed to help him to use what he has in order to effect a livable relation with his everyday realities.

Rank, who made a lasting contribution to modern psychological thought, gave a clear appraisal of the essence of therapy when he said: "Allow the patient to understand himself in the immediate experience which permits living and understanding to become one where, for the first time, we find a striving for an immediate understanding of experience, consciously, in the very act of experiencing." [8] He further states what Meyer emphasized: "The value of the therapeutic experience like that of every real experience lies in its spontaneity and uniqueness." [9]

The individual may be, and usually is, caught in certain patterns of behavior that have developed in the course of previous living. The truth of this statement is self-evident. But it is what the patient can find in himself and in his present relationship to bring about alteration in these patterns that interests the therapist. He is concerned with change and accelerating the individual's capacity to bring that about, with helping him to find *he* can change and not *be changed.* He will realize that the anxiety and antagonism stirred by the process of taking help may lead to an initial distrust and avoidance of self-initiated steps by the patient. He will know the significance of the patient's attempt to project on him all the impetus for change in order to struggle against the therapist's efforts to bring this about. The therapist must recognize that his skill and training have no therapeutic value unless they are *used* by the patient. He will have to know that the past holds a quality of safety and protects the in-

[7] Meyer, Adolf, *op. cit.,* p. 23.
[8] Rank, Otto, *Will Therapy* (New York, Knopf, 1936), p. 38, and the entire chapter "Past and Present" (ch. 4).
[9] Rank, Otto, *op. cit.,* p. 9.

dividual from the more pressing realities of the immediate hour. He will know the significance of the patient's use of past experience, both as it contributes to his use of this new experience and to the content of it. Putting this knowledge into action will enable the patient to move toward a real use of this therapeutic experience to evaluate himself more truly in the realities of the present.

The past is distorted when an individual attempts to use it to avoid the present, which is reality. We see examples of this all about us, as in the daydreamer who avoids life by making the present a dramatized past. Drama utilizes this human tendency, often poignantly, as in Thornton Wilder's "Our Town," where the girl who has died is portrayed as resentful of death and insistent on recapturing a moment in her past life. The attempt is a barren and disillusioning stepping back to a previous present, which has neither meaning nor reality as it is brought again into existence.

Theorists, in the attempt to explain the present by tracing everything back to a particular past, itself once present, say this or that is why we are acting in such a manner now. They tend to overlook the fact that when the individual reactivates the past he is doing it in a present which gives that past a new meaning which never belonged to the original set of events or feelings. In addition, this emphasis implies that the individual cannot be responsible for his present behavior because of the operation of unconscious forces over which he has no control. Thus when a child embarks on new therapeutic experience, he may react with the fears and anxieties that constitute in a measure the problem for which help is sought. But the growth-inducing values do not lie in uncovering past causes and orienting these new feelings to such events and attitudes. The new emphasis centers about what he can begin to do as these anxieties are stirred in this new relationship, and in how he can acquire attitudes about himself that will enable him to be free of these disorganizing feelings. When he finds he can live through the fear roused by this new reality he has begun to travel the road toward greater freedom to be himself. And the only thing a therapist can do for anyone in a therapeutic experience is to help that person gradually to be himself, to help him gain a sounder evaluation of his own difference and the consequent freedom to make creative, responsible use of that difference in the continuing realities of his life, whatever they may be and wherever they may occur. This is the measure of a healthy individual: free to live in each new present and to borrow from previous presents the stuff that gives continuity to life; and free from a past to which the neurotic is too tightly bound.[10]

The dynamic value of the immediate experience is to unburden the individual from those parts of his past which for him were destructive, and to help him affirm certain positive values in that past which he may have denied. One important medium through which that is made possible is the therapeutic experience emerging in the present the therapist and patient build together. The therapist has no actual connection with any other part of a person's life, even though the patient may "tell him everything." The very telling gains therapeutic meaning not merely for what is told, significant as that may be, but by the fact of the patient's acquiring a freedom to tell and to share. This is important for therapists to bear in mind when they are inclined to place too great therapeutic value on their interpretations.

Some historians have arrived at a similar evaluation of past material and have seen how false and misleading certain

---

[10] Rank stressed this point when he said: "The neurotic lives too much in the past and to that extent he actually does not live." Rank, Otto, *op. cit.*, p. 39.

deductions may be when present facts are explained historically. In an earlier article I [11] referred to the work of Teggart and would like to quote again from him: "Preoccupation with original documents brings with it a sense of security, a conviction that work based on primary materials must be necessarily sound and enduring. Hence the academic historian holds to the belief that having discovered the facts all that remains to be done is to state what he has found without prejudice or bias. It is not to be wondered at that, having adopted this view, he should be non-plussed, and eventually irritated, when it is pointed out that the end of this effort is the composition of a narrative marked by partisanship and emotion." [12] Teggart goes on to state that "the contrast between the acceptance of the 'present' as a situation, emerging as a result of antecedent actions, and the 'present' as a condition of things, resulting from operations of changes in the past, reveals the source of all the difficulties and differences of opinion which have arisen in dealing with history as a subject of study and investigation. History as an academic subject deals with situations and happenings, with actions and motives, not with the problem of change and not with the processes through which institutions, arts and ideas have undergone modification in the course of time. As a consequence, academic history ends in narratives which embody, for each generation, the human interest of the past, not in statements as to 'how things work' in the world of men."

In thinking of these statements in relation to human development we are confronted with some thought-provoking parallels. For a therapist to know all about what has hap-

[11] Allen, F. H., "Therapeutic Principles Applicable to Work with Children," *American Journal of Psychiatry*, v. 94, no. 3 (November, 1937), p. 673.

[12] Teggart, Frederick, *Theory of History* (New Haven, Yale University Press, 1925), p. 25 and p. 75.

pened in the individual's life history would be to provide him with an interesting historical narrative. But the therapist is concerned with the problem of change and this narrative leaves him with a cold set of facts, not with a picture of a present living person who has sought help in order to effect changes he cannot achieve alone.

Some child guidance clinics still operate on the assumption that there is value per se in accumulating "complete" histories, and base this assumption on the false belief that if enough can be learned about situations and happenings and motives change will take care of itself. Or they believe that a person can be changed by the "complete understanding" a therapist acquires through having all these facts. It is the actual reality of the troubled parent and his disturbed child and not the historical narrative per se which holds the central interest in therapeutic work. The healing values inherent in the present experience in which therapist and patient meet are sidetracked and even lost when we overlook the present and follow only the tortuous and endless task of trying first to evaluate all that has preceded. To understand the present, even though its content may be largely in past terms, is our major therapeutic responsibility, and from that understanding can emerge, actually, a better evaluation of the past.

A brief illustration taken from a complicated situation with an adult may make this principle clearer. Toward the end of a series of interviews, the patient told of a conversation with a man who acted as though he knew all the answers, who could be told nothing and had a ready explanation for everything whether it concerned him or not. The patient went on to describe that same quality in himself which previously had seemed to him like strength but which he then could see as a protection against the dangers of admitting any limitations. In the man he described, he saw and understood the ghost of his previous self. He could understand the past now because of his movement away from it.

These basic principles emphasize the utilization of the differentiating values that grow from the immediate therapeutic relationship. Here the therapist is a participating influence in changes that the individual initiates and carries on in himself. The therapist is enabled to do this because of certain distinctive features that make this relationship different from the others of everyday life. When we ask ourselves what constitutes this "uniqueness," two elements, already mentioned, return to the foreground. First, it is a relationship sought by the person who needs help. He acts because of the need to effect changes in himself. Second, the therapist accepts the responsibility of offering the help that is sought and sets about to participate in the building of a relationship that has a particular purpose and ends with its achievement. The function of this relationship is dually determined: one needs help, and the other is there to meet that need.

The main point I would emphasize, however, is the living nature of the experience. A relationship between two people is its foundation. Naturally certain techniques and skills are required, but we have gone far beyond seeing therapy as the application of techniques and the giving of insight. That day is over. If this relationship does not embody the elements that make of it a living experience there can be little therapy. The patient is, as I have said, a human being who must find new values in himself, not in isolation, but in the relation with another human being. This is the living element in the experience, and takes it beyond mere technique and explanations. Suttie states this clearly: "Therapy deals not with ideas and their logical arrangement but with free emotion of an unpleasant character or with its inhibition effects such as loss of interest, seclusiveness, etc." [13] While in essential

---

[13] Suttie, Ian D., *Origins of Love and Hate* (London, Kegan Paul, 1935), p. 204.

agreement with this, I would go further and add that the positive character of emotion, so frequently disguised by or transposed into unpleasant emotions, is as important in therapy as it is in life.

Since the therapeutic relation embodies the elements of a living experience, feeling is an essential part of it. By feeling I mean here the quality of a human being that makes him more than a biological mechanism, that makes him a living, related, functioning person. There is no life that exists apart from life. No human being can live entirely to himself. It is impossible to envisage a biological phenomenon, in this instance a human being, having an existence entirely its own. Child has stated: "Every biological problem involves finally all of life and the environment of life," (p. 5) and he further adds: "The organism as a pattern, a mechanism has no meaning except in relation to environment." (p. 7.) [14] He subscribes to Spencer's definition: "Life is the behavior of protoplasmic systems in relation to an external world." (p. 11.) These truths serve to re-emphasize here that the essential dynamic in all living is contained in relationship with others. As I have said elsewhere,[15] it is the universal fact of difference that makes a relationship possible, and, even beyond this, it is the reality of difference that makes life possible. A plant establishes its difference from the soil in which it grows. By a process of give and take the balance is established that enables the plant to grow and yet, at the same time, preserve its difference from the soil. Through living, the individual establishes his own sense of difference from the reality in which he lives. As the child grows he becomes more aware of his difference, and from this fact spring both satisfaction and suffering.

In the first chapter, the family was discussed as the institu-

[14] Child, Charles M., *op. cit.*, p. 5 ff.
[15] See Chapter I.

tion in which human differences are defined and given meaning through the roles of father, mother, and child. All of the clinical problems in child psychiatry involve, in some measure, turmoil that stems from difficulties in defining the interrelated differences in these three roles. Individuals in difficulty seek help to solve these dilemmas. With this step the therapeutic experience begins. It is a heightened and deepened experience in living that constitutes the heart of therapy.

In Chapter I, considerable emphasis was given both the principle and the process of differentiation as it occurs in the normal growth process. The same emphasis is in any consideration of the therapeutic process. Differentiation, by its definition, involves the formation of units that have their separate existence and function, while maintaining a relation to the original source of life. Child [16] made this clear when he emphasized that differentiation and integration are parts of the same process. Cells divide and new cells are formed, but these can exist as separate and functioning cells only as they maintain their relation to each other. The same is true of the integrated aggregate of functioning cells called a "human being," who acquires his capacity to function and develop not by isolating himself but by maintaining his new connection, both to the original source of his life, and to other humans who enter his horizon as he grows.

In the therapeutic experience the same principle of differentiation holds true. In his difficulty the patient comes, or in the case of a child, is brought, to the therapist with whom he has no previous relationship. But the fact of coming to a therapist, with all the feeling crystallized by that act, brings this new person into his life in a way unlike that of any other human relationship. Immediately, the therapist stands for a great deal. He may represent the source of salvation and the only hope of the future; or he may stand as the great danger

[16] Previously quoted in Chapter I, p. 19.

who possesses the power to do for the patient what he cannot or will not do for himself. The child usually will respond
to this new situation in a manner characteristic of the problem for which help is sought. He may be fearful or aggressive, demanding or placating, silent or overactive, and so on.
Whatever the response, the feelings awakened are now experienced in the relation with a therapist, who is thus brought
at once into a highly significant connection with the child's
turmoil.

How a therapist assumes responsibility for himself is of
great importance in this experience. While the patient uses
him in a variety of ways, the therapist, from first to last, must
maintain his own integrity. It is the therapist who provides
a steady background, through his acceptance of the patient's projections without, however, becoming in actuality
what the patient tries to make him. The patient, whether
adult or child, may use the therapist to symbolize the more
unacceptable parts of himself, may see in him his "bad" self,
or the "perfect" self he is vainly trying to become; or he may
attempt to place the therapist in the role of the mother or the
father with whom his relationship has miscarried. The skillful therapist will be fully aware of the importance of these
shifting roles assigned to him, but at the same time will
clearly know the necessity for preserving his own integrity
amidst the patient's veering about. In the therapist's role is
the firm backlog for differentiation as the patient perceives
his growing self as separate, as well as related, and as he has
less need to use the therapist to affirm this feeling.

These general therapeutic principles accent the value of
the immediate experience and apply whether the patient be
adult or child. However, therapeutic work with children has
certain unusual features which require special emphasis. The
child, unlike the adult, is still in the process of growing up,
and his emerging self has the quality of incompleteness and

of greater dependence upon others, particularly upon the parents. The problems that stem from the growth process, as most problems in children do, cannot be understood solely from the child's reactions, nor can a full knowledge of the attitudes and prejudices of the parents provide sufficient understanding of the difficulties. The problems, as I have said, exist in the relationship between parent and child. The self of the child is not to be understood in isolation from the other persons who represent so much that is necessary for his existence. This is an established psychobiological principle.

Earlier efforts in therapeutic work with children centered chiefly on these parental and environmental influences. The child was hardly seen at all as a participant in his own growing up. This one-sided therapeutic approach viewed growth as something happening to or done to a child. Change in the child was believed to be possible only if attitudes and events determined by others were modified. In clinical work this was a period of long records, with frequently meaningless details of developmental history, followed by carefully planned "recommendations" as to what parents or others should do to bring about happier conditions.

Equally one-sided were the therapeutic efforts that centered altogether on the child and neglected the fact that the parents, contributing also to the problem, must have a real and participating part in therapy. If everything is focused on the child it is as if he were only a biological entity, and all the causes of the difficulties lay within himself. The parents are expected and allowed to do little, aside from being "cooperative," and bringing the child at the appointed time. If one works with the problems as they exist, neither in the child nor in the parent but in the relationships which parents and children have together, the therapeutic effort has a different wholeness and balance. The very structure of a child

of the problem. They come together to the waiting room. The child may have been prepared by explanations of one kind or another about the clinic or he may have been told little or nothing as to why he is there. Both parent and child may be quite frightened, and that feeling may be openly borne or disguised in devious ways. They have embarked on an undertaking of considerable significance in coming to the clinic at all, and in taking this step together they are giving open recognition that the problem that requires help exists not solely in the child nor in the parent but in the relationship they have together. In the living drama of the first separation in the clinic waiting room the whole problem may be revealed, as child and parent experience the varying degrees of fear and resistance so closely related to their difficulties.[18]

Thus, the first seeking of help by the parent, and the subsequent coming together of parent and child, with the separation and reunion that takes place, has in it the essence of the entire therapeutic process. If no positive significance is attached to parent and child reactions to this structure of working, the direction and meaning of the whole experience will be altered. For example, if the fear that is set up in a child by coming to the therapist is seen principally as a barrier to therapy, to be removed by reassurance or by interpretation in order that therapeutic work can begin, the direction will be quite different than when the fear is seen as the first evidence that something is beginning to happen between the therapist and the patient. Real help can be given to the child by understanding his need to be afraid, and by supporting him as he finds what he can do with that feeling in this new experience. The same is true of the resistances set in motion by coming. If they are to be "broken down"

---

[18] More detailed discussion of these reactions characterizing the beginning hours will follow in the next chapter.

before therapy can begin this is very different indeed from a therapeutic approach in which the resistance itself is accepted as containing, at its root, the very strength from which a new feeling about the self must stem.

This way of working precipitates a variety of responses which the therapist must be prepared to meet, not historically but in terms of their immediate meaning. He must be ready to utilize whatever it is that the child brings to this essentially novel experience, to start right where the child is and build with him a relationship that is to result in eventual self-definition for the child.

Psychotherapy with children usually is initiated not by the child but by the parent. This fact alone constitutes an element not found in adult therapy. Some therapists regard this as a barrier to getting started. Sometimes it is, but more frequently this fact sets forces in motion that make therapy possible, particularly if the therapist is skillful in making use of the responses that crystallize around this and give meaning to the step forced upon the child.

The fact that the child is brought to a clinic may serve as a threat to him, which rouses both fear and resentment. This is particularly true if the parent, in bringing the child, is able to let the child know some of the reasons for a step which implies or openly recognizes dissatisfaction with the way the child is behaving, and asks that he change. Being brought to the doctor specifically for this implies to him that he is going to *be* changed. When he arrives, he meets this strange unknown force and goes, usually alone, to a room where child and therapist are together.

No human being, whether child or adult, wants to be made over by forces outside of his own control. The individual naturally guards against the impinging of forces from without, designed to bring this transformation about. It is natural, therefore, that a child comes organized in some

degree *against* the implied and imagined power of the therapist to effect change with or without his participation. The
child begins by marshaling his forces against this strange
person. These forces, accepted and understood, represent
the strength of the child to defend his own integrity. They
may be the very reactions that have created turmoil if the
child has been struggling with realities that have required
change which he has stubbornly refused to accept. He meets
this new experience in the same way, but in thus meeting it
he is at least putting his own feeling into it. He may passively
sit back and, by doing nothing, try to isolate himself. He may
be overtly fearful or antagonistic. In any event, he is responding with forces that are his own and in doing that much
he has become an active participant in eventually bringing
about the change which, at the moment, he may be fighting
against. This is because he finds a person who will respect
and understand his need to feel the way he does, a person
who does not begin at once to try to change him, but who
is concerned with the way he is feeling about being there
and about the reasons that have brought him.[19]

These reactions are not to be regarded as preliminary to
the therapy which can proceed only as they are cleared up.
Such a view would regard therapy as a process that is brought
about rather than as an immediate and continuing process
which happens and grows out of the shifting realities of a
new relationship. That it is unique quickly becomes apparent to a child who, at an impasse with the demands of growing up, comes prepared to struggle against this fresh force
that he feels as a supplement to those he has been fighting
already in one way or another. For a child to be accepted as
he is, is quite unlike his other experiences. The child may be
accustomed to struggle from long use, and here, instead of

[19] For an illustration of this statement see the first interview of George
in latter part of this chapter.

finding a person who gets involved with his struggle, he finds one who can help him express his feelings openly.

But the realities of this experience soon bring about fresh sources of turmoil. Certain conditions define this relation. The child has an established time during which he is with the therapist and separated from the parent (usually the mother). There are limits to the way he can live out his feelings, because the therapist will maintain his own integrity and define certain rights of his own. The child can feel angry but when he wants to destroy or attack he will find a person who can stand steady before that force and set bounds to his action. If he wants to play he has certain materials available which he may use or refuse to use, depending on what he is ready to do. If he wants to talk he has a ready listener who is interested in what he has to say. He may come, as one child did, with the avowed determination, "I won't tell that man anything," and find himself talking freely through his own wanting to and not because of any subtle or applied pressure.

It is important to consider, at this point, the value of what children tell about themselves. My conviction is that the therapeutic value of talking lies less in the particular content and more in the freedom to talk. Talking is a sharing medium, a means of communication between related individuals. A child who has gained freedom to talk, whatever the content, has gained a freedom to share himself. A child who is determined to share nothing of himself finds it necessary to continue, in therapy, the same guarding against getting involved in a relationship with another person. The therapist can meet and help with the feeling back of these reactions, and continue to respect the child's need to reserve some of his secrets, whatever they may be, for himself. The therapist who is preoccupied with eliciting a particular content, who leaps with eager zeal to each word connected with

move toward taking back into himself that which he thus disowns. Illustrative material concerning this will be given in subsequent case discussions. The early projections serve frequently to break up the child's complete feeling about himself, e. g., all "bad" or all "good" and the step is a necessary and potentially positive one. But it loses much of its positive value if the child, with the skillful help of the therapist, cannot reincorporate a new balance in himself, a part of which he had to project.

A ten-year-old described this movement succinctly. He was a boy with many fears which he had found useful in maintaining an undifferentiated relation with his mother. She had been caught in the web of these fears and found her life revolving about efforts to reassure him and to make his life more secure. Considerable progress had been made toward a freer and surer acceptance of his own individuality when he remarked: "When I first came here I thought the most important thing was to get things out. Now I know the important thing is to get them back in me." The first step was projection, in the form of talking and putting his problem out where he and the therapist, with whom he had become identified, could work on it. In this experience he began gradually to move toward a recognition of his own difference and separateness. His need for the therapist lessened as he became a person in his own right. He was able to take back, as his, that which he could own and use. This boy put into words the heart of the whole process. But he could not reach the second important stage until he had differentiated himself from the therapist who helped him first to project and then to reincorporate in the new self that which was emerging out of his therapeutic relationship.

All children, as they grow up, gain a sense of their littleness in relation to those who are big. But for every child there is some conflict over big and little that defines the difference between child and adult, particularly in roles of parent and child. A three-year-old boy, at the end of a period of therapy, stated this difference quite clearly when he said to his mother: "Mommy it's all right for you to tell me what to do because you're Mommy and Daddy, but when I grow up I'll tell myself." This conflict is commonly encountered in therapeutic work with children. The therapist either becomes the big, protecting and all-curing person in whose arms, figuratively speaking, the child can safely rest and do nothing, or he becomes the powerful person who is met or matched by the strength the child can muster to overwhelm his power. Thus he makes himself big, and the therapist small.

These are descriptive terms that the child uses as he accepts or attempts to deny his difference from the therapist. It is by means of the projections and the testings that continue through many therapeutic hours that the child begins to arrive at a perception of the worth of what he really is. Big and little are found to be not antagonistic, but capable of existing together and on friendly terms. The reality of difference between child and adult is found to be a livable reality. Only then can the child make creative use of his strength. Otherwise his effort will be expended in matching and overcoming the power that impinges from another, and, in so doing, in trying to deny and avoid the positive value of what he has and is. If the therapist emphasizes his own determination to help and strives to mold the child into the pattern of his choice, he complicates the therapeutic situation by becoming, actually, the force which the child tries to create in his own projection. This "therapeutic urge" can block therapy. Taft refers to this when she says: "Intention, or too often, determination to help is as poor therapy for a child as for an adult. It relieves the other of all responsibility and permits an unlimited negative exercise of the own will." [20]

In each therapeutic hour many opportunities arise for giving meaning to the reality of difference between child and therapist. Limitations enter naturally, and there are opportunities for the child to take responsibilities he might otherwise try to avoid. "You tell what I shall do today" is a common formula of the child who is fighting any responsible use of himself, as is: "I am going to stay ten minutes longer," or, "I will not put any of these things away," or, "I want this toy and I am going to take it." Limitations must have more than restricting or negative value if they are to be of help to a child. They provide the basis for definition of the nature of a relationship, and animate the reality of what is going on. A skillful therapist has no interest in proving he can make a child put away his playthings or clear up the mess he has made during the hour. He will not use the setting of a limit for the exercise of personal power. To do that would be to destroy the meaning of the whole experience, and make it the battle of wills the child may want. Valid limits grow from the situation and belong to it. They do not spring from the personal whims or control of the therapist. Around the natural limits that emerge, a therapist, by clearly defining them, helps the child to face them or to express his feeling about them.

Whether or not projection, as it occurs in the therapeutic experience, will be utilized positively depends upon the point of view and the skill of the therapist. If the therapist gets caught in the verbal content [21] of the projection he may

---

[20] Taft, Jessie, *op. cit.*, p. 110.

[21] The word *content* covers a great deal. The term has been used here to refer to topics of conversation, descriptions of past and present events or phantasies in which the child is describing verbally events, people, and himself and, in fact, to everything the child says. In a broader sense content refers to feelings that are experienced around what the child is doing or

miss the essentially dynamic quality in the use the child is making of him. What the child is actually doing and feeling is more significant than the verbal content that describes what he is doing and feeling. Hence the child may talk with the therapist about anything he chooses, to convey the feeling of what is happening in his relationship with the therapist. He may put considerable force into maintaining himself on the basis of his projections, or he may use play as the medium and symbol for his feeling. The important thing for the therapist is the maintenance of a sensitive awareness of what the child is doing *now*.

Through the child's reactions in beginning therapy,[22] an important principle in therapeutic work comes into operation through the skill and understanding of the therapist. The therapist will know that he is powerless to effect a change in any human being, child or adult, without the participation of the individual in that change. He is there to give direction and meaning to the changes the child can begin to effect in himself. He provides a medium in which change can take place and is not the force that demands or makes it. All the explanations and interpretations that the therapist gives do not, in themselves, bring about change. It is the child's new experiencing of himself, with a person who can accept him as he is, that gives clarifying value to these interpretations.

Many of these theoretical problems require illustration and discussion through the use of case material. Some repetition occurs, of necessity, as the value of play, the dynamics of the beginning and ending phases, and specific responses in therapy will be dealt with in greater detail in separate chapters. Actual case discussion brings out what is important in a

saying. In this sense a child may say nothing in an hour, but there still would be a significant content.

[22] Illustrative material on the beginning interviews is discussed in Chapter IV.

prise. The variations in response to this first separation experience in the clinic will be discussed in greater detail in the next chapter. But enough has been said about the dynamics of growth to indicate that this new experience takes on unique value and gives an immediate connection between what parent and child are beginning to do and the problem that has brought them. With this introduction, we can now consider the movement of George throughout a series of seventeen treatment interviews.

In his first hour George was quite guarded. His earliest reaction was a mixture of fear about leaving his mother and going with this new and strange man, and a timid friendliness toward the object of this fear. His first conversation brought in his father and the new automobile, bought to replace the old one which "isn't any good any more." He saw some toys and tentatively said, "I like your toys," and agreed he would like to play with them. But he was not going to move too fast, so added, "I will play with them a little while and then I will go home." George was proceeding at his own pace, and this was appreciated by the therapist, not in words but in his unobtrusive friendliness which could allow the child to evolve slowly his own reactions to this new person and situation.

In the course of this hour he explored the room, and was intrigued with each new thing he discovered. But frequently he said, "I always go home," or, "I will show this to my mother." He began to wonder where his mother was and had the impulse to seek her out, but when he was told that we had a certain amount of time together and then he would go home with his mother, that was enough so that he could stay for his full time. This was no mere reassurance, but served also to give more definition in time to this experience with the therapist.

The anxiety became more apparent, however, when

George said: "I haven't seen my mother since I came in here. I had better go now. I have played long enough." There was open recognition of this anxiety in the therapist saying: "George, you are a little scared of being in here with me." The important thing was that he could be that afraid without having everything revolve around that fear. When the therapist made no move actually to go to find his mother, George was able to stay.

At the end of the hour when we met his mother he said to the therapist: "It was nice to meet you." "It was nice to see you, George. You will be coming to see me again." He was intrigued but uncertain, and added, "Don't you come to me at my house?" "No, you will have to come here to see me." In leaving he waved and said, "I will see you sometime."

This first hour contains many of the basic elements of a therapeutic experience. An anxious, controlling child was struggling against the separating reality of growing up. A mother trapped in her own uncertainty and too great sense of responsibility was unable to give any realness to the mother role. Both were caught in a growth dilemma. The anxiety that had locked these two people together destructively was activated again in the child's first therapeutic hour but now with a person who was able to help him admit his fear and to begin doing something about that fear. It is true that there was little verbal content that connected this fear to his past life, and therefore no delving into causes by reaching back into that past. Indeed, the opposite was true. The interest and focus were on the present, living boy, and on the feeling content of the hour. It was the immediate experience that brought into the foreground the disturbances of feeling that made help necessary, and enabled this new relationship, even in one therapeutic hour, to take on significance for both boy and mother.

The same guarded and self-reassuring manner again was apparent a week later when he said, upon seeing the therapist: "I will come and see you a few minutes and then go home." That made staying, and his wanting to stay, a little safer. He proceeded to use this hour to differentiate himself from his brother and father. It was his first step towards gaining a clearer conception of himself in his relationship with the therapist, and it was fascinating to see how he used people in his own family as the medium for this. Referring to his brother, George said, "When Bill will be a big man I will be big too, but Daddy will be bigger. Once I was a baby."

George recalled the therapist's name and timidly indicated his liking to come. He was not so frightened in this second hour. He referred frequently to the old car and new one, and still held to the idea of having his mother come to the therapist's office. He recurred to the question of size, and of his relation to his parents: "My Daddy will bring me when I get bigger," and then made his younger brother bigger than himself, finally reversing the order. The conflict between his big and little self was out in the open. His relation to his mother held his feeling of littleness, and this was threatened by his present experience. At this point, George again became worried and said: "I have been seeing you enough. I don't want to see you again so I guess I'll go and stay with Mother."

There was far less fear in this and more of the little boy's determination to cling to the control contained in his fear and in his littleness. He was more determined to have what he wanted than he was afraid, and he found, around his desire to go, a chance to struggle and be more assertive. The therapist was the "bad man" for not encouraging him to go, and with a flare of bravery George asserted: "I don't like you. I want to stay in my house." Yet he made no actual attempt to go although he was relieved when the time was up.

In his third hour, there was more of his desire to go back to the mother. The therapist's office was still a dangerous place, and was definitely associated with bigness. He talked about a big boy who hits little boys. "Big boys are bad. They break things. Sometimes I have to do what Billy does." Bigness and badness were associated closely in his feeling, and he was seeking for a symbol to indicate that feeling about himself. For the first time he showed more direct interest in his therapist: "Where do you live? Do you have children?" and, "Do other children come here? I don't want any ladies to come in here, only boys." Suddenly, in the midst of this, he stopped and said: "Now you call the lady and say we are ready to go." He did not have to insist on this and at the end of the time he said: "I want to go out alone." As George left he smiled a good-by and called, "I'll see you next week."

In his fourth hour George was aware that something important was happening, and was much more disturbed. It was harder for him actually to leave his mother and the minute he was with me he asked: "You will let me go, won't you? I want to go when I am finished. I will go when my mother is finished. Then we will go home." The anxiety which originally was aroused by leaving the safer haven of his mother for the strangeness of a new experience was now being reactivated around his being engaged in this new adventure of self-discovery. As he began to acquire a more mature and growing feeling, he was more aware of what he was giving up. In the midst of this hour, which was a hard one, he started to paint, and, in the release that followed, George said with greater confidence, "My mother calls my daddy 'Daddy,' and I am George, and Bill is my brother, and I am bigger, and I will be a big man some day." The therapist gave support to this new awareness he described and through which he was discovering his difference, and George added:

sion of feeling, and centered the projection of his "badness" on the therapist. He used whatever he could to do this. He used occasional note taking and the therapist's pipe to give reality to his projections. Under the protection of this projection he was assertive and bossy and commanding, wanting to keep all the control in his own hands. As George was talking about badness, the therapist said, "You are talking about George." "No, I'm not, I'm talking about you," he replied. Then he returned to the role of a doctor who deprived his patient of desserts, put him to bed and said to the therapist: "You are going to be sick." The therapist commented: "And you are going to cure me." "Yes." But George, in the role of doctor, had his patient grow worse!

In the next few hours George maintained vigorously the projection of his own aggressiveness. Acting on his assertion, "You are bad," he intensified his "curative" efforts. Occasionally he became too actively aggressive and the therapist had to limit the expression of this. The controls which George knew were there and which he could depend upon made it safer for him to be aggressive. He did not have to bear the whole burden of limiting the expressions of his feeling. The comfort of authority is real in the life of a growing child and when the therapist (in this instance) set a limit, the child frequently showed real relief.

In George there was a close connection between fear and badness. In the midst of making considerable noise he said to the therapist: "You are scared, you are a bad boy." The aggressiveness continued, and the therapist had to limit its concrete expression: "George, you feel as bad as you want, but there are some things you can't do." George was both angry and anxious and said, "You shut up. I am not bad. I don't want to be bad." But it was important for him to discover he could feel angry and want to be bad, yet accept some limits as to what he did with that feeling. Until that is discovered, there can be but little emotional growth in any child.

In the twelfth hour there was an interesting and significant shift. He announced at the beginning: "I will make a mess. You sit down and write." Making a "mess" with paints had been a favorite medium for expressing his aggressiveness and the taking of notes was one of his justifications for making the therapist the bad person. Now he was beginning to accept some responsibility for what he did, and at the same time he could allow the therapist to have his own activity. The therapist was less necessary as a projection and became more of a real person as George himself became more real. It was the natural sequence from the preceding therapeutic hours and it was also George's first indication that he was approaching an end to the therapy. In that same hour he sensed that, as he talked about the end of the school year, and said that next year "I am going to another school, a big school." To the therapist's comment, "You are getting big," he smiled and replied, "No, not yet."

There were five more visits after this. These were characterized by a mixture of gentleness and assertiveness. The assertiveness had a more natural, less strained quality to it and the gentle friendliness in this boy came out spontaneously and without the fear of his losing himself in it. There was further discussion of his family, but with greater assurance of his own identity in the family group. His activity turned toward making things, and away from the more aggressive "messing things up."

In his thirteenth hour George and the therapist settled on termination to the therapy. This came easily, as he was free to let the therapist see that he was about through. His desire to leave early had little of the anxiety that characterized his earlier desires to escape. Now he really felt like leaving, and when the therapist said, "George, you are about through coming," he simply said, "Yes." Then he added, "Bill [his brother] will see you, he has never seen you. Can I go now?" He was using his brother as a symbol of his little self which he was leaving with the therapist as he was assuming the role of his more growing self. (In the final chapter of this book the dynamics of the ending phase of therapy will be discussed in more detail.)

George's ending had significance in terms of his growth in this particular therapeutic experience. He was sensing his own difference from the therapist. When he asked, "How old are you," he brought out his own age and feeling of bigness. He was accepting his own bigness in contrast to the bigness of another. In other ways he differentiated himself. He asked, "Have you a grandmother?" and when he was told "no" he grinned and said, "I have a grandmother and a grandfather." But he could not let it just stand as difference and added, "We have a new Ford, maybe you have a car just like ours."

Ending was not easy for George and roused the anxiety that customarily belongs to this phase of therapy. Once or twice he tried to extend the time, and in his last hour he went back to some of his insistence that the therapist was bad, and found it hard to admit his own apprehensiveness about the ending. Then he began playing with a cigarette and put one in his mouth. For him that was a daring thing to do. He watched closely for a reaction and when nothing was said he smiled and put the cigarette down. He had set his own limit. After a moment the therapist smiled and said, "George, you want to be like me in some ways." He relaxed and gently said, "I want to grow up," and could now agree that that was happening.

In the last few minutes of his final hour George repeated his question about the grandmother and emphasized that he had something the therapist did not have. Then he took some paper and handed over a piece saying, "Here is your ticket, you go on the steam train." Right at the end of the hour he took a piece of paper himself and said, "This is for home." With the poignant simplicity of a five-year-old child, George thus brought to an end this intensified growth experience.

This case has been discussed in considerable detail in order to bring out the importance of the process of therapy, an understanding of which can be utilized to invest with meaning what a child does in this new experience. In coming to the clinic and in establishing this relationship, a relationship in which an eventual termination was implicit from the beginning, we have all the important elements of a therapeutic experience. With George most of the feeling and verbal content belonged to and was aroused by what he did in the hour itself. He talked about and used outside people and events to give more definition to his own changing feelings about himself. When George and his mother finished treatment they left as mother and child, in contrast to the undifferentiated quality that had previously characterized their relationship. She had restored in herself the values of being a mother. George accepted being a five-year-old child. They were ready to resume their growing relationship together.

This case gives one graphic illustration of how a child and a mother change through a therapeutic relation, and it is from the understanding of this that the principles defined in this chapter have emerged. The theory I have presented here has not developed abstractly. Instead, it stems from the recognition of what people can do about themselves within the framework of the helping process. Human beings cannot be squeezed into the restricted boundaries of a theory and then made to serve as proof of its validity. The theoretical part of this book grows from an appreciation of the dynamics of human growth as I have seen that happen, again and again,

more uncertainty. Whatever the response, it is soon clear that this first step is of prime importance for them.[1]

As a next step in treatment parent and child come together. Sometimes the parents have prepared the child with a frank discussion of their reasons for bringing him to the clinic and have indicated that all of them need help for their mutual difficulties. Other children are told nothing but are just brought. Others may be told about the "nice person who plays with little children." Some may be fooled in more evasive ways, and many are told: "I am taking you to a man who makes children behave." Irrespective of the explanations given, the fact that the troubled child is having to face a new situation will leave him wondering and anxious about what is going to happen to him. That is inevitable. The child himself has not been the one originally to seek help, and being brought into active participation in the experience now crystallizes for him two important implications. One is that he needs to be changed. Irrespective of whether the preparation has been clear-cut or evasive there is in this step the implication that change is necessary. The second and more subtle implication is that the child is to have a part in the procedures designed to help him with his difficulties. The very fact that he is given his own separate appointment with the therapist implies that he has something to do with his own growth, that as he has been a participant in the creation of the problem, he now can be a participant in effecting change.

The important thing here is that the actions and attitudes of the adults concerned seeking help with the child and the responses of the child that are brought into play by this step

[1] For fuller discussion of the significance of the parent's step in seeking help and the part the parent has in the therapeutic process, cf. Almena Dawley, "Interrelated Movement of Parent and Child in Therapy with Children," *American Journal of Orthopsychiatry*, v. IX, no. 4, October, 1939, pp. 748–54.

give particular significance to the first interviews with both parent and child. They arrive at the clinic together for their first appointment but go separately to their interviews with therapist and case worker. At the end of the interview they meet again, and leave the clinic together. This may seem like a routine procedure and, in itself, to be of no particular meaning. But the responses that frequently appear may be dramatized expressions of the problem which has necessitated this step. The fear aroused in the child and the anxiety of a parent who trusts her child to another person and allows him to go with that new person without the support of her presence is not incidental behavior requiring only a reassuring tone or word from the therapist. These are reactions that precipitate the therapist into the very heart of the child's emotional turmoil.

The child is embarked on an experience which awakens feeling he must immediately come to terms with. He may be afraid, or may be angry or defiant, or he may be just passive and indifferent. Whatever the behavior, the fact that he is responding with his own feeling and in his own way makes him, from the very outset, a participant in an experience that will revolve and develop around his feelings. He is immediately placed in the center of a relationship that is significant because of its uniqueness. It is unique because he finds a person who is able to accept him just as he is. If he is angry, he can be helped to experience the full surge of that feeling. If he is fearful, the child has the support of a person who can understand his need to be afraid and who does not immediately try to reassure him in order to take that feeling away. He comes expecting to be changed and ready to fight or protect himself against the power of this strange, unknown person. Instead, he finds a person who is interested in him as he is.

These are points which were emphasized in the preceding

chapter. We now see their practical illustration in the beginning therapeutic hours of a child who has been in trouble with himself and others and who is brought for help by his parents, who frequently start treatment with the same mixture of feelings he has. Irrespective of what the therapist does, children respond with feelings closely related to the difficulties they present. These will vary as widely as the types of problems and kinds of individuals who seek help. They occur at the very start irrespective of what the therapist does, since up to the moment of first coming together the therapist seems to the child a specter or a god, or a threatening and alien force with unknown potentialities. In that first impact the therapist now becomes a reality.

The degree to which the immediate behavior of the child is utilized in this beginning phase is influenced by the particular therapeutic approach. Only as these responses are understood in relation to the whole therapeutic process, and not as being merely preliminary to the therapy that will follow, can they be utilized for the growth-inducing values inherent in them. If the fears activated by the separating nature of this first step are seen as barriers to the establishment of a relationship, to be removed in order to reach other and "deeper" sources of fear, then the therapist will necessarily take more active steps to reassure the child and work toward the building of a positive "transference." Similarly, the therapist who holds that the antagonism and anger stirred in the child by coming for help are barriers to the establishment of a therapeutic relationship will strive as quickly as possible to change this response in order to inveigle himself into the child's confidence.[2]

When the emphasis in these early interviews is on the ther-

[2] For an excellent discussion of this use of the first interviews cf. Anna Freud's *Introduction to the Technique of Child Analysis.* Nervous and Mental Disease Monograph, Series 48 (New York, Nervous and Mental Disease Publishing Co., 1928), ch. I.

apist's activity with the goal of drawing the child into a therapeutic relation, the child's immediate reactions have a secondary place and are often interpreted as resistance. The point of view presented here and the case material that follows is the opposite of this. The child's immediate responses are the center of the therapist's interest. To help the child bring to this relationship his own feeling will be the immediate goal of the therapist. A child who can do this in his first hour may begin to find his capacity to express feeling, while at the same time making a connection with the therapist with his own emotional responses. This is an important step. There is no need at this point to delve into the hidden or original sources of the fear that may be stirred when the immediate situation brings the child face to face with fear and with the necessity to organize his own resources around that feeling. The therapist provides support for the child in his efforts to deal with the reality of this new experience. In doing this he enters into a significant and growth-inducing relationship with the child, a relationship which has a beginning and an end, with an intermediate period of self-testing and self-discovery.

The emphasis here is on the experience itself and not on the particular content of the experience. How the child uses this relationship is of more importance than what he says. A child may start by a frank statement of some of his difficulties and talk freely about what he thinks is the cause of them. The therapist naturally is interested in what he has to say and may encourage him to talk as freely as he will. But his major concern must be with what the child is doing with the therapist and the therapy[3] through talking, and with a sensitiveness to whatever uses the child is making of this. A child who

[3] In connection with this point I want to emphasize again what was said in Chapter I, that therapy is a precipitated growth experience, not apart from but akin to life.

part in his own development that sets the therapeutic process in motion. This is true whether the patient is a child or an adult. In the children's field this principle activates both child and parent toward achieving a different use of themselves to effect a sounder way of living. Both parent and child begin with the expectation of *being* changed. This is inevitable. It is equally inevitable that their resistance is organized against being changed by a force outside their own control. This is human nature. So, when they embark on this new journey and meet the individual who basically is concerned with their own potentialities for effecting necessary change, a conflict of forces is set in motion. With the child this struggle arises in a variety of ways in the beginning hours.[4]

The significant point is that this struggle gets under way in the first hour, even in the first moment. The seven-year-old child who, the moment he entered the room rushed to the toy shelf and announced, "I am taking this home," was not expressing a desire for a toy. He was using the toy as his first assertion of an uncertain strength which he had never learned to use constructively.

Only as the therapist can free himself from a preoccupation with all that has previously led up to these responses in other situations can he utilize the opportunity which therapy provides, and in the creation of which he has a part, to guide the child to a more valid use of his own strength in the subsequent therapeutic hours. Otherwise, he may not be aware of the importance of what is going on before his eyes, as he will be exerting all his efforts to entice the child into a relationship from which "therapy" is later to evolve.

More meaning can be given these general principles by illuminating them with illustrative material from the beginning hours of a number of children who have been brought

---

[4] One detailed illustration will be found in the case of Solomon in Chapter VI.

to our clinic for help. This material covers a variety of responses of children who, by behaving as they did, became active participants in a relationship that held potentialities for help with the turmoil which necessitated therapy.

A father came at the suggestion of the family physician to discuss the problem of his seven-year-old daughter, Sarah. It was interesting that he, rather than the mother, came for the initial appointment. The mother was more bound up in her daughter's problem and found it hard to face taking the problem outside of the inner circle of the family for help. The father described the fears his daughter centered about anything new, or about the anticipation of doing things by herself. This was particularly true of school. "Sarah never seems sure of herself and can always find reasons for not doing what other children are doing," he said. The father described her preoccupations with fears of sickness. Her complaints brought frequent visits by the family doctor, who usually found her in good physical health.

The first problem the father had to settle concerned the basis on which this child could be seen. In view of the child's fear of anything new, particularly doctors, he suggested that the therapist visit the home for the initial contact. Undoubtedly he was speaking, in part, for the mother whose relation to this child was quite protective. The child controlled the family by her fears. To have seen that child at home would have denied to the child an opportunity to do something about the fear that might be aroused if she were brought to the clinic. The father was told of the clinic's way of working. It was discussed with him that, since the child's fears necessitated their seeking help, it seemed important not to protect her from whatever fear might be aroused by bringing her to the clinic. If the therapist had gone to see the child for the first visit they would have begun treatment on a false basis. He would have assumed, as the parents had, the child's complete powerlessness in the face of her fears. Fear represented this child's rigid control of her own growth, and might have become her control of the therapist had he gone to her. She had set up her own terms for growing, and this represented the stalemate and constituted the problem. The father and later the mother, who came for one interview before the child's interviews started, were able to accept the value of this way of working.

When Sarah and mother came together for their first appointment, both were quite frightened. The child clung tenaciously to the mother, who tried in an ineffectual way to reassure the child. The fear of the child focused on two immediate decisions required by the situation. First, she was afraid to come into the room without the mother. This was the separation fear which was at the root of so much of her trouble, and it was precipitated around the necessity for her to go alone to a room with a therapist. In addition, she was faced with the necessity of allowing her mother to leave her and go to another room with the social worker. The fear served the double purpose of keeping the child from taking this first step in the new growth experience, while, at the same time through her fear, she controlled the mother and kept her from leaving her. The child's use of her fear was partly effective during the first hour, as the mother did not leave the waiting room. She sat there and let the child find out for herself what she was ready for and could do.

Sarah stood in the open doorway, undecided whether she would come any farther. She could see some of the play material in the therapist's room and was obviously intrigued. The therapist commented that there were things she could use if she wanted to come in. She was interested and asked where they were. When the therapist told her, "Over there in the corner," which was out of her range of vision, Sarah gave up her uncertain struggle and came in. Sarah agreed she had been afraid of what would happen to her and for the fifteen minutes that remained she presented a mixture of a relieved but still rather tense child.

On her next visit five days later the performance of clinging to her mother was repeated. There was, however, a difference in both mother and child. Sarah announced, challengingly: "I will only come as far as the door." She was told she could come as far as she wanted to, and no issue was made of it. Clearly there was less fear and more open determination in her behavior today. The mother then turned to the social worker and quietly announced that she was ready to go with her. With this she was ready to step out from Sarah's control, and Sarah protested vigorously. As the mother went ahead with her plan, the storm subsided. Sarah stood her ground, half in the door and half out. When the therapist said, "Why don't you come in, Sarah?" she answered, "Because I don't want to." This was evidence of real progress away from the fear so evident in the first hour. It was a more open and responsible acceptance of her determination which no longer required support by fear. She was nearly ready to do something different, and a few moments later came in to the therapist's room of her own volition.

In this material we see how the clinic's way of working assumes a dynamic significance in the child's basic problem. Sarah and her mother, locked together in a relationship with little satisfaction for either of them, found they could begin to do something to break that up. Both had opportunity to feel just as afraid as they actually were, no longer needed to be protected from the reality of their own feelings. At the same time, Sarah did not gain control over this new experience by the use of fear. This was but the beginning of a

As a result, he was unable to keep friends and was heart-broken each time they left him. While he had a strong drive to give to others, he found it hard really to take anything from anyone. On each birthday he was critical of his presents, and frequently had nothing to do with them until several days had elapsed. This difficulty in taking from another person created a severe educational problem to the extent that he appeared retarded in all his subjects, particularly reading. Learning at school required that he take both instruction and direction. If Bob gave evidence of having learned something, he could never admit that anyone else had been involved in teaching him, and he usually minimized the value or meaning to him of whatever he was doing. He had to be in control. To take help from another person involved a recognition of another person's difference, a differentiation of himself as a person.

The relationship between the mother and Bob was an unusually close one. She was a widow and it was necessary for her to work. Each morning Bob would say: "I know you have to go but I wish we could have today together." The mother felt the strength and need of this attachment for herself. It was not easy for her to seek help. But she was ready for a different kind of relationship with her boy, and she realized that seeking help was not solely to enable Bob to be rid of his fears; it was a step in helping him to gain a self. The boy also seemed ready for change within himself, and when he was told about coming to the clinic he seemed quite eager.

Bob had heretofore used his relationships with friends and family as a means of denying his difference. He needed to absorb them, to incorporate them as an undifferentiated part of a self he could not accept as his own. But there was no security in this way of living, as he was threatened with the loss of all he tried to gain. In consequence he had no friends, and this reinforced his need to hold on to the mother. In this he had her encouragement, since the mother depended on the boy almost as much as he did on her. But to maintain this closeness in living meant that neither mother nor child could fulfill their real roles; he could not be the boy he actually was, and she could not be the mother. These roles defined the very differences neither could affirm.

In the classic case of Hans, the five-year-old child discussed by Freud,[7] there is an illustration of this same problem. Hans was enmeshed in the same growth dilemma as was Bob. He had little certainty in himself and was fearful of his emerging difference from his mother. In his friendships he tried to maintain that sense of ownership and used the pronoun "my" when referring to them. To like another child was synonymous with possessing the child. Hans, just as did Bob, suffered a tremendous sense of emptiness and loneliness at each successive loss of a friend who could no longer bear this great absorption.

This brief statement of the problem may be sufficient to give meaning to Bob's first interview, and to point the way to seeing how quickly this new experience became related to his whole growth problem. The mother came with him and introduced a tense and determined boy who acknowledged the introduction by grabbing the therapist's hand and vigorously pulling it up and down. This aggressive and possessive act served to cloak the fear stirred by the step Bob was taking. By his handshake he seemed to take possession of the new person, and entered the room without protest. He stood in the middle of the office, with his feet planted firmly on the floor, and gave the appearance of being ready for anything. When the therapist smiled in a friendly way and commented he liked big handshakes, Bob blurted out:

[7] Freud, Sigmund, *Collected Papers* (London, Hogarth Press, 1925), v. III, p. 149–295.

"I knocked you down and I can do it again and I can bring my rope in here." These exaggerated assertions of his power thinly veiled his fear, which he was trying to disguise with his meager resources. He was scornful of the toys and all that he saw in the room. When he was called Bob he asserted: "Don't call me Bob." He insisted he be called Robert. Again the therapist agreed and asked: "Do you know my name?" He asserted: "I will call you anything I want." He could not allow the therapist, at this point, to be an individual. He also made it clear that all that he was doing was being done solely because he wanted it. The desire of anyone else was completely excluded. Following some relaxation from his first assertions, he started to play with soldiers, saying: "You be sure these are here next Thursday; don't forget, I am coming next Thursday." He was asked: "You think you would like to come?" and he again asserted: "You expect me because I am coming."

In the behavior of this first hour Bob was trying to establish and maintain control of this new experience. He made it clear that he was there entirely on his volition, and that he would allow the therapist to be an individual only on his terms. In keeping with this he let it be known that he would return, not because he wanted to nor because of anyone's desire, but only as the basis of demanding another appointment. To have allowed the therapist to be an individual at this point would have required far more confidence than Bob possessed. When he was asked what he thought of the plan to come once a week he said: "I came because I decided to. My mother did not know I was in the car." He then manufactured the story of getting into the car a half hour early, stating his mother did not know he was there until they were half way to town.

Some scattered play followed in this hour, and in this activity he manifested, in exaggerated fashion, the same need to own everything around him. The blocks were referred to as "my blocks." Ownership of the soldiers was assumed as they were made into powerful people who could do anything. One soldier could annihilate an entire army.

The opportunity for a clearer definition of the therapist as a separate person in this relationship came at the point of terminating the therapeutic hour. Bob was told he had fifteen more minutes to play. He flared up and insisted upon having forty-five more minutes, threatening, "When I am through you are going to have something to clean up." He watched for the reaction to this, and when the therapist smiled and said nothing, Bob smiled for the first time in this tense hour. When he asked, "How do you know when my mother is finished?" there was no doubt that his activity with the therapist had added meaning because his mother was with another person in a different room. The therapist brought this question back to Bob's immediate situation when he said: "Bob, I don't know but I do know when you will be through." "How do you know that?" he asked in challenging tones. It was explained that on each visit he would have forty-five minutes, and that he could begin now putting away his playthings because the time was nearly up. Bob scornfully added, "Is that so," and went on with his play. But shortly after this he asked: "How much more time do I have?" It was the first open indication that he had recognized some aspect of the reality which the therapist represented.

Around the natural limits inherent in this experience, the therapist had opportunity to give it real form, and to stand as a reality himself. Time is one of the important realities which cannot be controlled. A child can be belligerent in feeling but not in action. With this boy there was no need to limit the belligerent action as he was too fearful of his uncertain strength to do more than verbally assert it. The natu-

ral utilization of this time reality in the first hour gave form
and direction to the therapeutic structure and offered the
child a chance to find that he could actually take some direction from another person who was not the product of
his own will and under his control. This was a first step in
differentiation.

Bob continued to test out these new realities. After asking about time he said: "I think I will come here every day.
I wish I lived across the street." A comment was made about
his being a little upset because he could not come every
day, and he asserted: "But I can." No issue was made of this
and he turned this testing-out process to the toys. He saw a
bell and said: "This is my bell. I am going to take it home."
The therapist quietly said, "No," and Bob continued to assert his decision. "Bob, what you want you feel you own,
don't you?" was the therapist's comment, and Bob added:
"I get what I want. I will keep this bell."

It was clear Bob did not want the bell but he did want to
test out the therapist. There was a great deal of relief as he
sensed the therapist's strength. It made it safer for the boy
to assert and demand when he knew there was a limit outside himself which remained firm. He did not have to bear
the burden of living out the exaggerated power which he
was asserting. In finding someone who respected his right
to have power, however, Bob found that he could have
strength but could also relate it to another who, in some
ways, was stronger than he.

Bob maintained an easier tone in these final assertions. He
made a feeble effort to avoid putting his things away, but
when he was not criticized he proceeded to do it himself.
He maintained, nevertheless: "I will put these things away
the way I want to and the next time I come I will have a gun,
and I will crash right in and I am going to shoot you, and
I don't care. And when I get these toys put away I am going

to leave all by myself and if my mother is not ready I will come right back." Following this declaration he went to the waiting room alone to rejoin his mother. He was not ready for a more open recognition of what he had begun in this first hour. In these reactions around terminating the hour he tried to recapture the control which, during the hour, he had been able partially to give up.

The second hour, after the week's interval, continued the therapeutic process of the first hour. Bob's mother reported several of his comments during the week. He seemed relieved that he had begun treatment, and spoke of the therapist's room as having everything he wanted. He described the time limit as a rule that had to be respected. That evening, however, he was quite miserable and wanted a great deal of attention from his mother. Clearly he was deeply stirred by his first hour, and several times during the week he insisted that he be taken to the clinic.

In that interval Bob had wanted to buy a toy gun and his mother allowed him to do so. On the morning of the second appointment he shouldered his gun and announced to his mother: "Here comes my bad self." He showed some resistance to starting for the clinic, in order to make the mother assume more of the responsibility for his coming. This was quite a shift from his first unreal attempt to make the coming to the clinic entirely his own. He brought his gun and a mask, and as they neared the office he put on the mask.

When Bob arrived in the waiting room he was ready for anything: mask on, gun in hand, and handcuffs dangling from his belt. He acted the role of the bandit he pretended to be. The therapist commented: "Bob, you look dangerous today," and a smile lightened his tense and aggressive facial expression. He issued a challenge for a fight but when the therapist said, "I don't feel much like fighting, although evidently you do," Bob took off his mask, put his gun aside and asked if other kids had been in. "Yes, Bob, several have been in." Calling him Bob today stirred no protest.

Bob now announced: "I am going to make something, my mother said to." He could not accept the full responsibility for initiating this more constructive activity. He proceeded to make a sign on which was painted: "Keep Out." "And I will hang it outside and kids will think you put it there." To the therapist's, "Why don't you let them know it is your sign, Bob?" he smiled approvingly. He went ahead with his sign but found it hard to ask for help with it from the therapist. Instead of asking he insisted: "You are going to spell 'keep.'" He had assistance on this, but he did not respond to the comment about how hard it was for him to ask help or to admit that he needed it. Bob completed the sign, timidly opened the door and left it outside. His emphasis centered on the fact that he owned this place and was going to shut everyone out of it.

It was still necessary for Bob to test the therapist's ability to define the limits which gave a framework to this relationship. The boy insisted that he could break a piece of wood, and he was encouraged to try. He wanted more opposition however, and his assertion, "I am allowed to do anything I want," was really a question and a way of discovering for himself how safe it was to assert his power. He was not sure the limits he craved would stand. Children become frightened when, from the adult world, there are no controls set to their emerging sense of power. They need the steadiness and comfort of an authority which provide a backlog against which they can gain a sense of their own power. This is true for all children, but for this confused boy who needed so much and was able to take so little direction, the controls determined by the consistent strength of the therapist were essential. His dilemma was in his fear of a further loss of his poorly defined self if he accepted limits set by, or in relation to, another person. From this uncertainty his pattern was to control and not to be controlled.

At this point Bob was not sure enough of himself nor of the therapist to have any assurance of how the strength he perceived in the therapist might be used; nor could he be sure that it would hold steady and not melt away before his efforts to overwhelm it. When he stated, "I am the boss," he was testing out how far he could go in attaining that objective under the protection of the existing limitations, the nature of which he was gradually discovering. When he began to believe the therapist was not using these limitations to make him submit to an alien power he became bolder in his assertions of being the boss. He was finding a new and less total way of being the boss, and in beginning to make this discovery he was making his first differentiating step in his relationship with the therapist. This use of limitations highlights their real value in therapeutic work. They are never used in order to overcome a child's will; they are, instead, the means of helping him discover and use creatively a strength that can never have any actual creative satisfaction for him when it is used solely to conquer another.

At the end of the second hour Bob left his guns and mask and took only the handcuffs with him. It was as if this boy were leaving part of his "bad" self with the therapist. The feeling of "badness" in Bob was associated with his trying to annihilate totally the individuality of others through his efforts to possess them. In attempting this he was actually denying his own difference from his mother or the friends upon whom his forceful efforts were expended. He made a similar effort to destroy the element of difference in his first hour with the therapist. Through the preceding week the gun had symbolized both protection and a breaking up in himself of a quality that had always stirred fear. Whatever other meanings the act of leaving the gun and mask may have had, it was clear that Bob had now established himself in the new relationship, and the beginning phase was over. He was ready now to use the therapist to achieve a clearer perception of his own individuality.[8]

If we are concerned with the beginning phase of therapy as a part of a process of growth, we must consider the behavior and feeling responses that arise before actual contact is made with a therapist. The significance of starting treatment is revealed most clearly in some cases by what happens before the child ever reaches the clinic. In those parent-child situations where a deadlock has existed for a considerable period, much is already precipitated by the parents' reaching a decision to do something different about the child's behavior. Making that decision and acting on it immediately introduces a different quality in the relationship between child and parent, which in some cases of itself brings about radical changes. Miss Dawley, in discussing this point said: "With some children there is an immediate shift in symptom or behavior, occasionally after the mother's first interview and before the child has ever been in the clinic. If anything is to be done, he will do it himself." [9]

Such alterations in behavior emphasize the powerful effect on both child and parent of the step taken by the parent. The child may be precipitated into action, and the determination that impels him to act with his own resources is essentially a healthy thing. The difficulty with that type of change, however, is in its isolated completeness. In it there is lacking the connection between that change and a living reality which comes when change occurs in and

---

[8] The discussion of this case is continued in Chapter IX when the dynamics of the ending phase are discussed.

[9] Dawley, Almena, *op. cit.*, p. 749.

through a relation with another. Change thus emerges through a living experience, and not as a means of avoiding such an experience; it has, therefore, more stability.

This connection with a new living reality may be provided by the parent who, through the move of seeking help, indicates a readiness to assume fresh responsibility in his role of parent. This happens in the normal growth process. A parent will long tolerate a certain form of behavior, but finally reach the point of taking a firm stand. A child who gets more and more unreasonable in his behavior while the parent is trying futilely to "be reasonable" frequently settles down with great relief around a real and immediate assertion of feeling from the parent that does not have to be carefully thought out beforehand.

But in clinical work, where we often see the problem emerging from a tight, interlocking quality in the parent-child relationship, these sudden shifts occasionally encountered may need to have the stabilizing influence that comes from a therapeutic relationship that can continue even though certain behavior patterns have been eliminated. Both parent and child need help to consolidate within themselves this sounder organization of themselves. The following material will illustrate this type of change and the new quality that is frequently introduced into the first interview.

May, a girl of ten had maintained for years a severe eating problem. The mother stated there was no difficulty until she was four, when she began the refusal to eat. She vomited when forced, complained of a distaste for food, and had no appetite. Much time and money were spent on physical examinations. Various diets, tonics and medicines were prescribed, all requiring considerable effort from the mother. No organic causes were ever found. Once started on a regime which assumed a physical cause, however, this was maintained by the constancy and multiplicity of the child's

need to take me there, I am going to eat by myself.' " From that time on she ate enormous meals and on the day of the appointment May announced that there was no need to come at all as she had cured herself. The mother was wise enough to continue with the plan, however, and May came without protest.

This child, whose whole self had been engaged in this struggle over eating, directed that same determination toward assumption of control over her own change. If anyone thought he could change her she would fool him; she would do the changing! The child had sensed a real shift in the mother, which was represented by her coming to the clinic. Previous trips to doctors had been on the basis of the mother's anxiety. This was different; as implicit in it was the mother's determination to do something very different.

Naturally, the problem was just as real as before May started to eat, since her own change, up to this point, was actually her protection against being changed. But the first therapeutic hour set in motion some new responses. She stated her position by saying: "I have changed myself and therefore you have no need to change me." May had marshaled her strength against this new force that crystallized both the need of change and the fear of being changed. Then she found a therapist who did not battle with her but instead accepted her change and her strength for what it was. He did not see the change as resistance but as the beginning of a new sense of responsibility in the girl, even though it was too negative to be lasting. Yet it defined more clearly the therapeutic task. It was not to help the girl to eat but to help her to find a sounder and more lasting way of assuming responsibility for what she did that constituted the therapist's aim. He did not want to break down the new strength arising in this child; he wanted to help her make it real, to integrate it into herself, so that it might exist also, in new form, in relation to others. He did not want to let it remain as an organized effort to protect herself from being influenced by a force she could not control.

The therapist's capacity to accept the change for what it was, and not to make an issue of it nor to minimize its value, enabled this child to feel she wanted to continue coming. She had found her own desire and reasons for returning and thus made the coming her own. And in making it her own she was taking a step in differentiating herself from her mother upon whom she had previously fastened so much of the responsibility. The mother, who had carried that load, now was experiencing the anxiety of seeing the child herself begin to take over doing something about it. This left her puzzled, with a mixture of relief at seeing it happen yet, at the same time, a sense of great loss.

Naturally, May assumed that she was brought to the clinic to be cured of her eating difficulty. From her point of view an unknown and externalized force was to achieve this result. It was not the fear of change that stirred this girl into action but the fear of being changed, of having this done *to* her.

Another first hour will be used to illustrate a different pattern of behavior encountered in the early hours of a therapeutic situation, a reaction of passive guarding and non-participation on the part of the patient. The extremes of this pattern are found in the silent child, silent in words as well as in feeling, who shows no reaction around going off with a strange person, and may sit and wait for whatever may come. This child may be quite pleasant and agreeable and tell the therapist what a nice time he has had when he leaves, or he may use play as a detached medium for doing little or nothing that includes the therapist. Such a child presents a more difficult problem for therapy as he does not participate in starting anything. He tries to maintain an attitude that is neither for nor against the step he is being required to take by the parents who have brought him. Back of this need to hold to a neutral and nonparticipating attitude there is usually a great deal of determination, and the skillful therapist is gradually enabled to establish a connection with that force.

The child here used by way of illustration was not a completely silent child, nor one who lived so much in herself that the presence of another was but little recognized. Her pattern was one chiefly of indifference and passivity, and her behavior, in taking that form, indicated thereby the nature of her problem. Ann, a bright girl of eleven, does nothing in school. The mother, in describing this, said: "I am to blame for it." Evidently the child's passive pattern of living had been effective in placing the source of her difficulties outside of herself. She withheld her effort in a school psychological test to such an extent that the school questioned her basic ability. They were confronted with her apathetic attitude toward learning, and when the question of school demotion came up the parents were sufficiently startled to seek help. A psychological test at the Child Guidance Clinic showed that Ann actually possessed superior intelligence. In their relief at this, the parents had no incentive to initiate treatment, so that it was a year later before they really faced the problem of what lay at the basis of Ann's behavior. It was as if they could not let her have any responsible part in the problem. During that year the parents continued to urge and to reassure Ann, and each time any difficulty arose at school they would rush in and try to straighten it out. They blamed the school's teaching methods rather than Ann's passive attitude toward school itself. The final decision to bring the child for treatment represented an important step, in that it indicated that the parents finally had recognized concretely their need for help. In addition, it was the first real indication that they could let Ann have a chance to do something about her own problems.

At the time of the first therapeutic appointment Ann was slouched in a chair in the waiting room. She acknowledged the introduction to the therapist in her usual apathetic manner, and maintained an air of sophistication and purposeful indifference as she went with him. Her first verbal responses denied both interest and concern in coming to the clinic. "I never wonder or worry about anything. I take everything as it comes." She remembered her earlier visit for the test, saying merely: "It was in a larger room." This implied some criticism of the new setting but it also implied some of the anxiety stirred by being brought closer to her own problem. But Ann continued to insist that she had nothing at stake in this new venture and commented, as the therapist asked what brought her back: "I just came. My mother brought me and I am used to that." But the controlled effort to maintain her air of indifference covered the apprehension roused by this step, and made it necessary for her to do a great deal in this beginning hour. Ann's effort to do nothing started her in a direction that might lead to a different and more real participation if she continued. The therapist wisely refrained from precipitating issues but quietly maintained that since Ann was coming because of her difficulties, she had a real part in what might go on and maybe she had something to say about what her part might be. She introduced the subject of school, and said in an offhand manner: "I'm never interested in anything. I do too many things but I never finish anything. I'm not ambitious."

These were more than statements of a difficulty. Ann was throwing out a challenge, and using her problem to try to make the therapist take over the job of changing her and making her become ambitious. She was testing out this new person to see how much she could make him do. This was

use her ability. In this way she had made them assume responsibility for her ambition while she carried on the fight against it, and against them.

Ann continued to have weekly interviews for four months, and developed gradually a different use of her twelve-year-old self. The start she made in that first hour enabled her to use her relationship with the therapist to gain a more mature feeling about herself. Through the hours that followed she talked mainly about school and home, and emphasized in a variety of ways the irresponsible patterns of behavior which she was trying to maintain in her therapeutic relationship. The words she used referred to other situations but the feeling and effort belonged to the immediate hour. Through hours filled with uncertainty and struggle Ann had to find the kind of responsibility she could assume for herself.

Children are adept in creating, in their play life, imitations of what they want to be. They dress in adult clothes, they become Indians and firemen, and their play allows a dramatization of themselves in these roles. Dolls and other play materials are utilized to provide a structure for their "pretend" activity. Since play forms such a natural part of a child's existence, it is to be expected he will utilize it in the beginning hours, as well as subsequently, with a therapist. Some children come bringing their own play material to give an air of familiarity and greater safety to this new place.

I should like to cite, as illustration, one additional beginning hour of a child, who made interesting and effective use of her own material to initiate her relationship with a therapist, to round out this discussion of the therapeutic importance of the first hours.[10]

Patsy's father and mother had come, on advice of their

---

[10] A more detailed consideration of play as the child's medium of expression will follow in the next chapter.

family doctor, to discuss their worries about their five-year-old daughter, the second of four children. The child's difficulties centered about speech. She did not stammer but persistently used an infantile language of her own. Now that Patsy was in kindergarten, she was becoming sensitive about the speech which made her feel so different from the other children, among whom she could find no place. In her family relations she was tense, irritable, and exhibited many fears; and at home she was chiefly at ease with and related to the family cat. The mother's relationship to this child was a most protective one. Patsy had had considerable sickness, and this helped to accentuate the protective attitudes of both the mother and father. The mother had, by contrast, a satisfying and normal relationship with her nine-year-old boy.

Patsy had been told by her parents she was going to "see a lady doctor to see if she couldn't learn to talk better." Patsy seemed eager enough to come, and brought with her a favorite doll. Carrying this doll, she went, with apparent ease, to her first hour. She wore heavy glasses and her large muscular legs and awkward movements gave this five-year-old girl an odd appearance. The therapist stated her own name, and asked what Patsy liked to be called. Instead of giving a direct answer she turned to her doll and said: "She can talk. She can say Patsy sometimes, but she can't say you." The doll at once became what the child was supposed to be and what she was not ready to be in herself. When Patsy was asked how she felt about coming today she replied: "Ask Susie" (the doll), and the doll was then described as having some of the "scarey" feeling she had herself.

But Patsy did not need the doll very long. In her curious speech she said, "I can play," and soon she was engaged in putting blocks together in a house. When this play began she handed the doll to the therapist. "You can hold my doll if you want." There was real capitulation in this act and it had all the implication, in feeling, of the child's handing herself over to the care of the therapist. The house she built was a narrow aisle between two rows of blocks. The therapist said: "No one can get in that house." Patsy pointed to the small door adding, "No one big can get in." She agreed later, however, that some big person might get in. Then she said quite spontaneously: "I can talk."

This child had made effective use of a symbol of herself to take care of some of the anxieties of her first hour. With the increasing sureness she felt in herself, she gave the doll up and spoke more as herself.[11] No doubt she had done this same thing in many other new situations, and as an isolated experience this would have meant nothing. But here, at the outset of a therapeutic experience, it was the beginning of use of her own ability. In the hours that followed, Patsy made interesting use of the new experience to gain a better integrated use of her own capacities. The doll which at the beginning was a protection and a mask, and thus the means of avoiding her real self, was utilized by child and therapist as an aid for the child to come more into the open when she could begin to be herself.

Beginning where the child actually is and dealing directly and immediately with his feelings, rather than with his problem behavior and its causes, give an immediate impetus and meaning to the therapeutic process. The child is taken for what he is, and is not squeezed into any theoretical scheme nor cajoled into giving up any particular "secrets" or content. Whatever form the child's feelings may take, angry or fearful, happy or sad, aggressive or placating, talkative or silent, "co-operative" or "unco-operative," they engage the

[11] Oscar Wilde expressed this so well when he said: "Man is least himself when he talks in his own person. Give him a mask and he will tell you the truth." *The Prose of Oscar Wilde* (Albert and Charles Boni, 1935), p. 172.

therapist's immediate interest because these are the indicators of a troubled child floundering around to find a way of adapting himself to the world in which he lives. The child is accepted as having, within himself, the potentiality for achieving a new inner balance as he is helped to find value in a living relationship. Thus the therapist enters at once into a significant relationship with the child and becomes a growth-inducing influence throughout the steps that follow.

These beginning hours with the child must be understood as an integral part of a therapeutic process and not as preliminary to it. They are as much a part of therapy as dawn is a part of the day. Any therapeutic philosophy which fails to catch the significance of this and neglects to utilize the feeling responses aroused in the child by starting a new experience will miss the opportunity to give this new experience immediate significance in terms of the turmoil that requires therapy. If these early responses are seen as preparatory, it implies that therapy is regarded as springing from the therapist and from what he says and does. If therapy, however, is viewed as a child-centered experience, then whatever reactions the child brings can be used to aid the child in achieving a new sense of himself. This can never occur in isolation. It must occur as a living experience. It is that which begins in a variety of ways, in these first hours with a child who, because he is confused and troubled, is brought for help.

found entirely in the specific situation the child relives. There is more than incidental importance in the fact that the child's responses take place in a situation in which he is also engaged in active relationship to the therapist.

Here I shall approach the problem of the use and value of play from a broader viewpoint that centers the emphasis on the nature of a child's activity as he participates in building a therapeutic relationship. Since play is his most natural medium for the expression of feeling, this form of activity inevitably is of primary significance. The focus of attention is not on the particular type of play but on the spontaneous responses of the child through play as he relates himself to a person who is prepared to help him over some of his difficulties.

The word "play" carries for most people a meaning synonymous with pleasure or having a good time. As a result, when the word is used in connection with therapeutic work with children, this common impression comes to the fore, and the child is pictured as just "having a good time." This may be a particularly disturbing impression for a parent who brings a child to a clinic because of an accumulation of irritations and difficulties and then discovers that the therapist allows and encourages him to play. A natural reaction of some parents is that the child might instead have gone to a neighborhood playground, or have stayed home and played with his own toys. Why go to the trouble of bringing him all that distance to a clinic, and pay a fee when "all that he does is play."

These are some of the reactions to a word that connotes pleasure. Most people think of work and play as opposites and sometimes envy children who spend so much of their time at play. But, for a child, play is so much more than

restored their confidence. Allison, George F., *American Weekly*, as published in Philadelphia *Record*, April 21, 1941.

pleasurable activity. Children quickly sense this in the therapeutic hour. A child of six who started a serious battle between the "goodies" and the "badies," which clearly represented his own dilemma, turned to his therapist and said: "I'm not just playing." In his everyday life play is the child's natural form of expression, a language that brings him into a communicating relationship with others and with the world in which he lives. Through play he learns the meaning of things and the relation between objects and himself; and in play he provides himself with a medium of motor activity and emotional expression.

Therapy must occur within the framework of a relationship that is established through the participation of two people. The child, as one of the participants, may and frequently does find that play activity is the natural means of bringing something of himself to this new experience. The therapist cannot establish a relationship with a child who does nothing any more than a child can find a connection with the therapist who is passively inactive. There must be a mutual give and take. Everything centers about the child in this particular relationship and he must be helped to use freely his most natural medium to bring to this new relationship his interests and feelings. So there is no mystery to the fact that children are provided with an opportunity to play in therapy. Only through such activity can the element of naturalness enter in. If the parents are ready to accept the worth of the child's participation in the step they have initiated by bringing him for help, this explanation of the special meaning of play will be sufficient. If they cannot face the importance of letting the child have his part of the problem, then their irritation, which actually has little or nothing to do with the pleasurable reactions to play, will continue. Helping the parent to deal with these questions is part of the other side of therapy which is not discussed in this book, but it must be constantly kept in mind as a significant part of the process which this book attempts to describe.

It is the uniqueness of this relationship and of the circumstances that bring it about that give special meaning to what the child does, whether it be playing or talking or just sitting. The child is in trouble and he is brought to be helped. This move, as I have already indicated, stirs up feelings that are closely related to the trouble that makes help necessary. Whatever the child does in this new experience is colored by these feelings. He needs a medium of expression to organize and objectify these feelings. Some children, particularly older ones, can do that in words. Frequently, however, even older children also need and use the play medium. When a fourteen-year-old boy noticed the toys in the therapist's room and scornfully said, "Those are for little kids," he was coming closer to his own dilemma. In his feeling about himself he partly wanted to be the little boy he scorned in his false efforts to deny these feelings with this fourteen-year-old status. Later, when he gained greater freedom to be what he felt like being at the moment and played with some toys, he was taking a step toward using this new experience to harmonize the attitudes he had over "being big" and "being little." As he was able to accept a more mature status, the nature of his activity in the therapeutic hour changed.

The therapist who bears these points in mind will be less concerned about initiating any particular type of play activity. He will be interested in helping the child do whatever he is ready to do, and will assist and encourage him in choosing what actually is valid and useful for him. Frequently, a child may be blocked in finding his own medium of expression by the urge of the therapist who is too anxious to get him to do some particular thing. The child may be eager to play and may look at the toys with anticipation. But to start to play would mean yielding, and he may have come with the determination to do nothing. Too much urging of such a child at this point makes it harder for him to do anything but sit. The therapist's interest here lies with the child, with how the child feels, and not with rushing him into activity of any specific kind.

In the beginning, a child is told about the play material that is available for his use. Whether he decides to play or not, and with what materials, is much less important than the fact that there is choice as to what he will or will not do. He may dodge that responsibility and put it back on the therapist by asking: "What shall I do?" That may be a part of the child's timidity about taking any liberties in this strange place, or it may be the first evidence of a struggle to make the therapist carry a responsibility he will not assume for himself. Some children rush to the toy shelf and start playing at once, without any preliminary explanations, and thus try to shut themselves away from the potential dangers of this new situation. Others immediately find in play a medium for expressing the feeling that has been roused by this new experience. Other children may do these same things in direct conversation.

As the therapist becomes concerned with the various uses the child makes of play material to establish himself in the therapeutic relationship, he will be less concerned with the particular play activity chosen. With this orientation he can help the child to use the medium of his own spontaneous choice to experience and to share the feelings that have been aroused, and to take his first steps toward an organized and meaningful expression of himself in this new situation.

A child who is brought for therapeutic assistance usually is one who has been caught in some aspect of his growth toward a normally functioning self. Commonly, this means that he is unable to handle his feelings in a way that allows

phantasies operating in the continuous impulse to play," [5] he will utilize whatever play the child initiates in order to get at these hidden meanings, and will interpret them, as Klein suggests, "down to the smallest detail."

This is not the place to discuss these theoretical differences. I touch upon them only to emphasize that different uses are made of a child's play activity, dependent upon the point of view of the therapist. If he advances the last point of view stated he will attribute little value to the more immediate meanings of the child's participation in building the new relationship with the therapist except as they lead to a "transference" that will allow more specific content to emerge. But if the therapist is oriented to the primary value of the immediate experience he will be less concerned about the historical significance of what the child is doing. He will be concerned with helping the child to be what he can be in the here and now, and in assisting him to move toward responsible and creative uses of the self which has, to be sure, emerged out of the past.

Since play provides such an important medium of expression in therapeutic work, the setup of the office and the materials provided deserve careful consideration. Play material must be chosen to serve a variety of needs, yet too much material and too wide a diversity tend to defeat its basic purpose. Simplicity is the main consideration. A large place should be given to material that allows manipulation, both for destructive purposes and for creative activity. The aggressive feelings commonly encountered in therapeutic work with negative and anxious children require material that helps them to externalize and objectify these feelings in a play medium. Soldiers, toy guns, and similar toys offer material for aggressive expression and enable children to be

[5] Klein, Melanie, *op. cit.*, p. 31.

more daring with their feeling than it is otherwise possible.

We can see, from the following illustration, the use one child made of soldiers. A ten-year-old boy with facial tics was brought for his first interview by his zealous, over-responsible mother who had always guarded him from possible dangers. He was known as a "good and obedient child." In the therapist's office his attention immediately was drawn to the soldiers, but he would not touch them. Instead he went on to tell of his "bad" brother and emphasized his own "goodness." "He always wants my things but I never want his," was one way he disowned the bad in himself and kept only the good. Play with the soldiers represented a more aggressive and lively expression of himself than he could allow at this point.

During the hour he spoke critically of adults who "forget their promises." A casual comment by the therapist that boys also could be forgetful brought quick agreement, and he told of an incident when he went to the store and came back with the wrong thing. It was the first shift away from the unreal goodness he had been trying to prove. Immediately following this, he returned to the self-forbidden soldiers and initiated a vigorous war game. He had come to life and, with that, the facial tics, so prominent up to that time, temporarily disappeared. The soldiers were utilized to provide a concrete medium for feelings that had no chance of expression except indirectly through facial tics.

Children, with inadequate feelings of their power and fearful of what others can or might do to them, find in the toys associated with fight and aggression the reinforcements that they need. Just as a primitive can put a piece of iron around his neck to acquire its strength for battle, so can the child gain some of these feelings from the objects animated by his phantasy and need. Pliable materials such as soft clay offer an excellent medium for both aggressive and destructive feelings, as well as the opportunity for the child to build and create.

Dolls and household toys allow many children a chance for imaginative play that introduces the element of relationship, and these should be included in the play material. This permits the dramatization of a part of the self that is sometimes difficult to integrate into a livable and healthy whole. A doll or a nursery bottle is used frequently by children to represent the little or baby side of themselves. Such materials are used by children to externalize themselves in roles closely related to unacceptable aspects of themselves. For example, a child with enuresis first created that problem in the "dydee" doll, and then proceeded to punish and correct the doll for this behavior.

Less desirable are those toys that allow little opportunity for the child to modify them and mold them according to his need and feeling. Mechanical toys and complicated puzzles have little use aside from momentary amusement value. When there is a tendency for the child to become so absorbed in the thing he is doing, the fact that he is doing it with another may be lost. The activity comes to be too much of an end in itself. This is particularly true of complicated construction activities where everything centers on the thing being made.

Paints and drawing materials are most valuable. Particularly useful are the finger paints developed by Miss Ruth Shaw in her educational work with children.[6] This medium allows a child unusually wide scope for his movements. It is fascinating to watch a timid and guarded child, who is restricting all movement or expression, start with these paints, first with the tips of the fingers and then gradually extending his movements until one or both hands are making

---

[6] Shaw, Ruth, *Finger Painting* (Little, Brown & Co., Boston).

the broad sweeps that are possible. Children can put into a painting the feeling that cannot be given a verbal expression. While this material allows fairly wide scope and a chance for the child to "mess around," it is not chaotic. There are definite ways of proceeding, and rules which must be followed. Miss Shaw correctly emphasizes a regular procedure of wetting the paper, covering the whole paper with the chosen color and cleaning up after the painting is completed. Around these rules the child may struggle vigorously, and through such activity gain some recognition of what he can and cannot do.

Occasionally there is a place for such games as checkers. This may offer a child a familiar activity which he can carry on with the therapist. It may offer a timid child with few resources an opportunity to do something with the therapist, as in the case of a twelve-year-old girl who found initiating anything almost impossible. This fitted in with the selfless quality that characterized her problem. It seemed important, in this instance, to set into motion some activity, even if initiated by the therapist. She was not a negative child but one who seemed utterly helpless. She accepted a suggestion that we play a game of checkers, and through this activity the first hour ended with a more animated quality in her. In the next hour she was able to initiate a little activity of her own, and it was not checkers.

The primary principle to keep in mind is that what the child is doing is less important than his freedom to do something. A wide variety of toys is distracting and makes play in itself such an intriguing and absorbing thing that its main therapeutic purpose is lost. In the playrooms that are equipped with fascinating toys and a wide variety of things, we may see a great deal of activity but little therapy.

Play materials help many children to bridge the gap between the new experience and their more familiar everyday

of the experience are diminished by a too active assumption of the various roles the child will assign him. This does not mean, however, that the therapist becomes a passive observer. Play offers a chance for the therapist to be a part of what a child is doing without becoming just the object who fits into all the child's desires. Usually this is accomplished by a sensitive interest that responds to the child's comments and feelings; and joining him in those activities where he can maintain his own identity.

These general comments about the child's play activity need to be pointed up in concrete case material that reveals children in the actual process of beginning and carrying through a therapeutic experience. The meaning of what I have said previously will thus become clearer. I have selected the case material which follows as illustrative of the nature and purpose of the child's activity, and of how the child's play changes as he moves along through the differentiating steps of his relationship with the therapist.

Mike, a seven-year-old child, was brought for help by his mother. His problem could be summed up around his having so little sense of himself. In school he sat and participated hardly at all. His entire development had been slow. "He is like somebody lazy," was the description given by the mother, who felt he was bright enough but was making little use of his ability. During the mother's first visit to the clinic Mike waited passively in the reception room. Before the mother's interview was over he came to the door and announced his presence by a very gentle tap on the door. He was near tears, but he took a small toy offered him and sat in a little chair. Toward the end of the interview he was included in the conversation, and was asked if he would like to come to see the lady who would save time "just for him." He smiled and the mother, a simple but genuine person, said: "Mike, this will be your first date."

In his first hour, alone with the therapist, Mike made feeble efforts to smile but he was closer to tears. He sat in the same chair he had used a week earlier, and looked quite frightened.[7] In a casual but friendly manner he was told where he could find toys but that he might need a little help in opening the door of the toy closet. Instantly he got up and with some vigor opened the door. "You got it open the first time, didn't you, Mike?" He smiled and took a truck that had fallen out, but he had to be sure of the therapist's reaction to the noise before going further. He was told that "when the rest of those things fall out they will make a big racket." He proceeded silently to take everything out. They talked about the trip to the clinic and how he came this morning and Mike told, with his infantile manner of speech, where he lived. Then he picked up some wooden pegs used to make animals and quietly asked what they were. When told, he left them in the cabinet and proceeded to play with the toy automobiles.

His interest centered on a drawer in the desk that was much closer to the therapist, and he slowly crawled over to explore. He looked at a few playthings but was afraid to touch them until he was told: "You may take out any you want, Mike." While he gently moved a few toys the therapist took one of the crayons and casually started to draw. His attention was drawn to this and he said: "Making a house," but went back at once to his toys. Gradually he drew closer and closer until he was practically under the therapist's chair.

Suddenly he looked up in distress and said: "I'm poopin'." He had soiled himself and was taken to the toilet. The mother was called and helped him get clean. When he re-

[7] In this case the person who had the first interview with the mother continued with the child. While this does not usually happen, in this case it was felt necessary because of the importance of what had been started with the child in that first hour.

turned to the office, he came up to the therapist and whispered: "Something happened." The therapist, sensing his deep disturbance, met this reaction in a friendly way and rightly assumed some of the responsibility by saying, "Yes, Mike, and now you know where the toilet is—I should have told you before." He played a little more, then said: "Pick things up," and efficiently put everything away. While doing this he was asked: "How about next week?" and his face lighted up instantly as he said: "Write my name." He silently smiled his good-by as he left with his mother.

In this hour a boy with so little sense of himself was making an effort to play with the toys which, if it had succeeded, would have represented a partial and purposeful use of himself. His efforts seemed only to draw his whole undifferentiated self into a closer physical contact with the therapist. The physical reaction that followed was an infantile reaction of the whole organism which was deeply stirred by the experience he was going through. But the simple meeting of the soiling and the therapist's sharing the responsibility for allowing it to happen, enabled him to have a real sense of being part of this relationship he was starting with another person.

Returning a week later, Mike's mother said: "He has been waiting for this all week," a reaction which surprised her as it was not like the passive apathetic boy with whom she had been living. He had begun to come to life.

In the second hour, Mike was, in actuality, the different boy his mother described. The moment he entered the room he made a spontaneous dive for a toy gun. The therapist had made this available with the thought that he might need, and be ready for, a more aggressive and purposeful action. With great delight he shot the gun about twenty times, first aiming at the spot where another staff member stood just as he entered the room, and then at the spot on the floor where he had soiled himself the week before. He went from the gun to the saw and hammer and, with little need for encouragement, went ahead making a considerable noise. He was a better integrated child today, as was shown through his spontaneously chosen activity. In this setting he became more verbal and told about his baby sister saying: "I got a baby that big," indicating she was about a foot high. He had started to be a person and could begin to differentiate himself from another human being.

This rather poignant material illustrates better than any theoretical discussion the change occurring in a child's activity as he was helped by the skill of the therapist to use the material that was available to give organized expression to his feelings. In doing that Mike was taking his first step in becoming a person in his own right in this new growth-inducing relationship. He needed no reference from the therapist to the meaning of what he was doing in terms of his past, since he was engaged in the more important task of finding what he could be in the immediacy of this new and exciting experience.

The nature of the child's problem and the character of the relationships he has established heretofore naturally influence the activity he is ready to undertake in his therapeutic relation. The child who has had unsatisfactory or detached relationships may respond by sweeping the therapist into everything, or he may find it difficult to include him in anything. I shall present several illustrative interviews with a child of the latter type, a boy whose play phantasies were rich in detail but devoid of any real feeling. He was absorbed in the play activity which he described in great detail, and the presence of another person had, apparently, but little influence on what he was doing.

Bill was a boy with a strange background. His parents were well-educated and cultivated people and this seven-year-old boy was their first child. They were busy with their own adult affairs and the boy lived very much by himself for his first three years. The parents described him as contented in the isolation of his playroom, as from an early age he was quite ingenious in amusing himself. He was left to his own devices and received only the attention necessary for adequate physical care.

The arrival of a girl child was the beginning of trouble in the family, and brought the parents to a sudden awareness of their neglect. Bill began to attack the baby and for this he was punished. Thus a vicious cycle was established, which the parents were unable to break up. For the first time Bill was drawn into a relationship with his parents on the basis of his genuine feeling, and his aggressive, cruel reactions to the sister had to be maintained in order to preserve that relation. He knew no other way to have a connection with anyone. His antagonisms to his sister grew in intensity, and spread to other children. It was literally true he had no relationships that allowed either the giving or the receiving of positive feeling. Bill was a "lone wolf."

The boy was so disturbed that he could not be kept at home. He was placed in a small school, where he was when treatment was started. The parents brought him for his first interview, but after that they were not able to participate in the therapeutic work that followed. This undoubtedly influenced the long period of time necessary to help this seriously neurotic boy.[8]

Bill came to his first therapeutic hour without hesitation, and showed no evidence of being upset. Unlike so many children who start this new experience, he was leaving nothing behind and was separating from very little. In his man-

---

[8] There were fifty-seven interviews with this boy and they were spread over a two year period. There were two long breaks caused by summer vacations.

ner he was formal. His walk was stiff and his facial expression
flat and unrelaxed. He talked in a high-pitched voice, color-
less in quality and tone. He spoke mechanically, but without the coloring of a living and related child.

Without hesitation Bill went to the clay which he saw on
the shelf, and began to build a house. While he described
the detail of his activity, and seemed to be talking to the
therapist, actually he was talking into space. He used whatever material came within his range of vision. Blocks, sticks,
clay, paper, were thrown together in a heterogeneous mixture. It made no difference to him that the structure had not
the slightest resemblance to a house. His imagination made
it a house and that was enough, though it was necessary for
him to have material. The therapist's comments about his
activity and how he had felt about coming caused a momentary pause, but had no effect on what he did or said.
Bill emphasized the great strength and age of the house,
which was over a hundred years old. Then he changed and
said it was so old that it was crumbling and had the rain
wearing it down. Next a big storm came, and Bill proceeded
to destroy the house with the same meticulous care and regard for detail which went into its construction. No one
lived in the house, it was as devoid of human contact as was
this boy. But a little fox, he said, had been caught in the
ruins. At the end of the hour he remarked that the house
was a thousand years old.

Bill's play activity, in this strange hour, so clearly revealed
the nature of this boy's self. He gave little evidence of real
aggression or anxiety in the new experience. Instead he
brought to the therapist the same unreal, unrelated quality
that characterized all of his living, as well as his play phantasies. Although he was only seven, he seemed as old as the
house he was building and destroying.

In the second and third hours he repeated the same activity, but with some differences. It was richer in detail and included "parent trees that had baby trees growing from the roots." Then a big storm came along that broke not only the trees but everything around them. Bill used both clay and the blackboard to dramatize the action of his phantasies. He missed no detail either in the drawing or in the verbal account, and his use of material was less heterogeneous than in the first hour.

It was in the third hour that Bill gave his first indication of being aware of living objects beyond his own phantasy life. He asked whether other boys came to the therapist's office and what they did there. Not only was this his first awareness of others, but it was his first question asked of the therapist who, up to this point, did not exist as a person to him. This was the first stirring of a more real quality in Bill. In this hour the house he built had people living in it. They were very poor people, and they all lived in one room with no flowers, and he described everything as "ugly." The family was asleep when the big storm came. "They are dreaming this is happening but they don't know it. They are still asleep and dying." He effected their destruction, saying at the end: "Now they are dead and in heaven." Bill's first talking about people had the same transient quality he gave the dream, as the hour ended with no life left in the characters of his weird phantasy.

In the third hour Bill saw a clay elephant left by another boy, and he centered about this all the phantasy in the therapeutic hour. This was as near as he had come to projecting any feeling onto a living symbol, and it was probably his first step in breaking up a total aggressive force in which his entire self was involved. But the projection of his badness [9]

---

[9] In this case material and in some that follows the terms "good" and "bad" have been used, as children constantly use these words, to describe

onto the elephant was so complete that it left no basis of connection with his own feeling. In an older person such a split might indicate a serious psychosis, and at times Bill presented that possibility. In these early hours the therapist could not touch him at any point that involved his own feeling.

Before beginning his own activity in this third interview, Bill asked many questions about the boy who had left the clay elephant, his age, when he came, and so on. Some factual answers were given to these questions, as the therapist realized that Bill needed an object invested with greater reality on which to project his aggressive phantasies. Ordinarily, questions of this type do not need factual answers as they indicate primarily the feeling and interest awakened in the child by the fact of his presence in the room alone with the therapist. A recognition of the child's feeling by the therapist is usually sufficient answer to the child's questions.

Now that the other boy was more real, Bill proceeded to remake the elephant, saying: "It is a bad elephant, he has never been trained." A wall was built around him and his trunk was stuck to the wall for punishment. He was moved to a truck which Bill sealed up so "the bad elephant will not escape." The therapist entered this phantasy play asking what made him think the elephant was bad. "He would not do the circus things right, they put him out." As he made the wall secure, he gloried in the heat created, told how

---

two poles of feeling and two sides of the self. Negative and positive have a slightly different meaning in that they refer to behavior reactions which may be felt by the individual as good or bad. The terms are not used with any moral connotation but more to designate feeling-tones which are harmonized in the normally growing child. The more neurotic child, who tries to achieve a more total feeling of goodness or of perfection, thus prevents the more alive and real balance that can admit and allow expression to the less lovely and good feelings as well. So it is also with the very aggressive child who cannot allow any of the more gentle and yielding and related feelings to be a part of his living. Such feelings indicate weakness to him and carry the threat of his being controlled by others.

"sweaty" the elephant was and emphasized: "This will keep him feeling bad because he has been bad," and, "This will hurt him but he needs it," and, "Now he is crying."

The therapist's comment that the time was nearly up started Bill on the intense destructive activity which ended each hour. While destroying the cage, he poked in at the elephant who "was all skinned up." "Now will you be good?" He had the elephant say "No" and then Bill slammed him on the floor. "Will you be good now," and a weak-voiced elephant said "Yes." Next the elephant was taken to the hospital where "he will get well and live happily."

Bill was completely absorbed in this vivid, aggressive play and the presence of the therapist seemed to mean little to him. He seemed hardly aware of a telephone interruption. Yet his vivid and complete projection of himself on the elephant had great meaning. He reserved all of this activity for his therapeutic hour. In his school there was no mention of these lively phantasies and he talked to no one about his visits to the clinic. He was always ready to come and eager to arrive on time. In school he was slowly adapting to the routine and, while he made no friends, he was making a little progress in his work.

The detail of the next hour showed how Bill was able to take a further step in objectifying himself in the medium he had chosen for his projections. He asked about the bad elephant, commenting: "He was nearly dead." The therapist referred to the elephant's decision of a week ago to be good but he overlooked that. Now it was a turtle that was bad, "A very, very bad turtle and he is going to be thrown into a well." The therapist asked what he had done. "He is not honest, he does not do the things that are right." It was fascinating to observe the rigid and moralistic attitude Bill took toward these external projections of his "bad" self, so split off from the "good" self he had assumed for himself in his play.

The therapist picked up a doll at this point, and asked if Bill had any place for it in his play. The therapist did this purposely, with the thought that Bill needed some help to bring his projections out of the safer realm of elephants and turtles. Bill quickly accepted the suggestion. "It will be a boy who will be bad. He is not honest. His name is Bob. He is nine years old." A jail was built. "No one will ever be able to get him out," said Bill. Asked the reason for his incarceration he quickly gave one. "He chopped a tree down. He will not get anything to eat and it will be very dark. He is much worse than the elephant, he is the baddest person in the world, worst in the last hundred years." Asked where his family was Bill told of his good father and mother who "think he should go to jail."

Bill continued with vivid details of cruel punishment, shutting off the boy's air, making it as "hot as fire" and knocking on the walls to scare him. Then he repeated last week's performance of asking: "Will you be good?" First the reply was "A tiny bit," and that led to more punishment. The second answer was a loud and vigorous "No." That started the usual destruction and the boy was "nearly killed" as the hour ended.

A week later [10] Bill announced: "He will be good today because he is afraid he will go to jail." He certainly was not letting the object of his projected badness move toward any real goodness. He again built a house, and described the inhabitants: "Very poor people live in it; they are cold and do not have enough to eat." Suddenly he changed them to rich people who live in a strong house, but immediately a strong

[10] This boy should have been seen at more frequent intervals than once a week, but arrangements could not be made to allow this.

bad he was taking a part of that feeling into himself. This was a natural movement on his part toward a more balanced feeling about himself. In a sense, Bill was doing the same thing even though he was further away from any readiness to feel any sense of ownership of the "bad," which he attributed to his play objects. But in taking for himself the role of the rigid moralistic person, who cruelly punished the bad elephant or the bad boy "the worst in the world," he was being the bad person himself in action, but with little responsible ownership of the feeling. When he could reach that point, at a much later period in therapy, the character of his hours changed completely. The destructive theme disappeared and Bill's whole interest centered around construction.[11]

The therapist's real responsibility lies in helping a child to do what he is free or ready to do, without trying to force him into any particular channel of expression. This is my chief objection to the more controlled use of the play as many therapists use it. Recently, a case came to the attention of the clinic where a six-year-old boy had long defeated a therapist's efforts to get him to use any play material. His determination was set against the determination of the therapist who felt that only in the child's play could he get to the "secrets" that the child held to himself. For six weeks the boy had successfully defeated these efforts, and never touched a toy. The family moved, and the child was referred to another therapist for help. This time the therapist was interested in the child and what the child himself was able and ready to do, and had no interest in getting any particular type of activity started. By the end of the first hour the child spontaneously began to make an interesting use of play ma-

---

[11] Further details about this boy are included in the chapter on ending (Chapter IX).

terial and from that point on was deeply engaged in his therapeutic relationship.

A common question raised by children in their early hours is: "What shall I play?" and a struggle may be set up in them against taking any responsibility for making a decision about that. Recently a boy sat for forty-five minutes, the entire time of his appointment, trying to make his therapist say he wanted to play checkers with him. That game had been played in two previous hours when the therapist had responded to the boy's partially expressed desire to play. In these hours his determination to act only with or through the expressed approval of the therapist became quite apparent. The therapist began the third hour with a casual friendliness but made no reference to what the boy might like to do. Abe looked at the checkerboard but took no initiative in asking to play a game. He fidgeted for a few minutes, then said: "I wonder if *you* want to play checkers?" The therapist asked in a casual way if that was what he wanted to do but Abe insisted that the therapist's desire came first, that he had no right to say he wanted to play. The therapist replied by saying that this was one place where he had that right if he was willing to exercise it, that it didn't make any difference whether we played or not, but all Abe had to do was to decide himself what he wanted to do. Abe kept the struggle going by saying: "You might not want to play," a risk he was not willing to take. This may seem like unnecessary detail concerning a minor point, but in this checker game, which by itself had little significance, an important reality in the therapy was being defined. There was no pressure to get Abe to do one thing or the other. He was allowed opportunity here to struggle to make another person responsible for his choice. His determination was engaged in attempting to force the therapist to make his decision; the therapist, on the other hand, was not forcing him to do anything. This made it possible and necessary for the boy to do what he actually did do, to sit and argue for that entire hour. But in the next hour Abe moved naturally into activity of his own choice, a move he would not have made if the therapist had fitted into his plan to avoid doing anything on his own initiative. This was a turning point in the case.

One more piece of material will serve to focus sharply a major emphasis of this chapter; that is, that play activity in itself has secondary therapeutic significance.[12] Meaning is given to the activity in large part by the fact that the child is building a therapeutic relation through what he is doing. This point becomes clearer in the following material where the participation was verbal, and there was no play.

Jane, a fifteen-year-old girl, lived in a small institution and was brought to the clinic because of her inability to conform to the group. Her temper outbursts and intermittent running away stamped her as a troubled and troublesome girl. In her first therapeutic hour she showed by word and manner her intense resentment at being required to come for help. The therapist met this reaction quite openly with her, and helped her to state exactly how she felt. The therapist said he knew the circumstances of her coming, but now that Jane was here he was concerned with the way she felt and whether she saw any need for coming. The girl, in tones that sharply indicated her antagonism, said that she knew she had difficulties but could see no sense in being sent to another person for help with them: "I can solve my own problems." The therapist understood this and brought out that seeking help seemed too much like weakness to her. Jane agreed instantly to this, and the therapist went on to say

---

[12] Play in the normal life of the child has spontaneous therapeutic value. I refer here only to the play activity in the therapeutic situation.

that it took real courage to face the fact with another person that something was wrong and that she was ready to do something about it. Jane reasserted that she could do that herself. The therapist agreed that ultimately she would have to anyway, and said that coming for help was not to shift that job, but to find more effective ways of doing what she herself wanted to do about her situation. Jane asserted the possession of three qualities: "Determination, pride and stubbornness," and the discussion was directed to the possible uses she could make of these potentially valuable traits. The therapist said that their value lay entirely in their use, and that evidently she was stuck in her efforts to use these traits in any constructive expressions for herself. She was directing them against other people, not for herself. The therapist suggested it was around a different use of these traits that he and she might get together on a helpful basis. The girl was actively engaged by this time and agreed, but reluctantly, that she might try coming a few times to see if it held any value for her. The therapist accepted this yielding but with the reservation that it meant more than coming and warming a chair. The girl was serious in her statement that she meant really to try.

Around yielding even this much to her own desire to change, there was a quick shift in the tone of the hour. Jane went on to tell of her early life, the shifting and unsatisfactory nature of her family relations, of her thwarted ambitions, and the mounting feeling that she was not necessary to anyone. The important thing lay not in what she told; the value was in her own yielding and in her freedom to share her problems with another person. She ended the hour in a relieved mood, and returned a week later with a readiness to participate actively. The fight against being changed was turned to a desire to participate in changing. In the interviews that followed, she accomplished a great deal.

Jane effected, in the more direct give and take of conversation, what another child might do in play. She began with negative feelings which the therapist accepted and used in this early phase of therapy. The child who uses play material can be helped to do the same thing with the feelings that animate that activity as expression of the meaning to him of the immediate experience. Each child or adolescent reacts in whatever medium he can, and the therapist's responsibility centers around bringing into the open the meanings that are there in terms of the only reality he has with that child, the present experience.

A clearer indication of the way this works out can be seen in examining briefly one complete case that covered thirteen therapeutic interviews. The illustrations in this chapter up to this point have shown the meaning of the child's activity in single hours, or in the early phases of therapy, but have not shown how the activity reflects the changes occurring within the child himself as the therapeutic process unfolds. When the therapist is oriented to the growth of the child through the therapeutic experience he will be able to utilize the changes in the child's activity to give impetus and support to the child's growth.

Dick was a boy of eight who had finally lost the uncertain anchorage of an unstable home and, at three years of age, was placed in a foster home where he was accepted as a "sweet, innocent little boy and loved very dearly." Actually he was an anxious and fearful boy, and the foster mother was drawn into a close relation with him through her desire to "give him security" and make up for the deprivations in his life. On the one hand were the great needs of the boy, and on the other, the overzealous readiness of the foster mother to satisfy these needs. The relationship that developed between them came without any effort on Dick's part, and he was swallowed up by it. His fear originally grew out of his having no anchorage in any relationship, but it was reactivated by the further loss of himself in the enveloping "affection" that centered about him while he was docile and sweet. The more acute fear, roused by this further loss of self in the absorbing relationship that was more satisfying to the foster mother than to the boy, led to such sudden and violent outbursts of aggression that it was necessary to remove him from the foster home. The foster mother could absorb the "sweet, anxious boy" but she had nothing to give to the fighting boy he became in her home.

The same sequence was repeated in two other foster-mother relationships until, in a final outburst initiated by an aggressive attack on another child followed by a resurgence of Dick's intense fear of dying, his disturbance became so sweeping in its physical expression that he was physically ill and was taken to a hospital. Thus Dick extricated himself from yet another relationship in which he felt trapped. Another temporary foster-home placement was made at the time he started treatment.[13]

From the history it was clear that Dick would probably begin his relationship with the therapist with the same feeling about himself that had characterized his previous relationships. In his first treatment hour there was an acute fear aroused by his having to leave the supporting presence of the social worker who brought him. She was his only anchorage. When he was told that his "visitor" would be waiting for him at the end of his hour, Dick cast furtive glances

---

[13] In the literature of child psychiatry considerable emphasis has been laid on "affect-hunger." More emphasis needs to be placed on the "affect-indigestion" so well illustrated in this boy. The well-intentioned efforts to satisfy Dick's need for affection served only to increase the need and the fear, because the inadequate feeling he had about himself made it difficult for him to feel any real connection with the sources of affection. This is an important point, not only in therapeutic work but also in the field of child placement. A too rapid absorption by the affections of a foster parent creates fear in a child.

at the toys on the open shelf and chose a gun which he timidly picked up. He was soon interested in arranging the soldiers in battle formation and talking about which side would win.

The play material offered this fearful boy an external medium of support while he was discovering who the new person was and what he could be with him. But in that first hour Dick could not really allow a fight to take place with the soldiers. There was too much fear for him to permit that much evidence of his own aliveness. He made it clear the soldiers were merely parading, and to make that even clearer, Dick mixed animals in with the soldiers, and a small doll who was "too little to fight." Simultaneously with this cautious use of material were further expressions of his anxiety about being with the therapist. "How long do I stay?" and, "Will my visitor take me home when it is time?" were questions that gave the therapist an opportunity to help Dick relate these fear reactions to the newness of this experience. The play with the soldiers continued, and Dick was intrigued with the possibility of a fight. He made preparation for this fight by placing the small toy figure of a nurse in the rear to take care of the people "who get hurt."

Dick's play reflected the same guarded feeling about himself in his second hour. He watched the therapist closely, and tried to make him responsible for each forward step. Cautiously Dick returned to his war game, placing the therapist on his side because, "We won't fight against each other." He could handle his own fear through his identification with the soldiers and said: "They are brave outside but scared underneath, and that is badder." Some support for his fear was given when the therapist commented: "We can all be a little afraid once in a while." When the child had the protection afforded by the fact that the hour was soon coming to an end, he allowed some actual fighting to enter into his play. Dick asked about time, and upon learning that three minutes remained, he asserted: "Now we are ready." In the brief period of fighting the baby was the first to get hurt. As the end of the hour was announced he said with obvious relief: "I didn't start soon enough. Next time we will have a good war."

Dick came to his next hour with greater eagerness, and started his war game at once. The therapist was assigned the role of the "big pig," and he took for himself the role of the "little pig." This was the first step Dick was able to take in differentiating himself from the therapist. While describing the support the pigs provided each other, Dick was able to allow "big" and "little" to enter in to his description of difference in his phantasy characters. Both pigs were placed in the rear line, although he said: "We are pretty brave." Dick gave the pigs the support of a cow because, "He is a good fighter, he has horns." After twenty minutes of anxious stalling the long-promised fight started, and in the ensuing battle all the casualties were on the opposing side. The pigs were kept in a safe rear position.

In the fourth hour Dick continued his slowly evolving war game. Again the enemies were annihilated and sent to the hospital where they were given care. The big pig was the aggressor this time. Then there was an interesting variation in Dick's activity as, for a short time, he left the war play. He took stamps from letters in the wastepaper basket, wanted the therapist to have his address and said commandingly: "You can write me a letter while the other children are playing in here." Dick had arrived at a point where he was aware not only of himself and of the other children who came, but of his desire to shut them out. It was his first direct assertion of himself. When he later returned to the battle activity, it had taken on a new significance, with the emotional and verbal content more directly related to this immediate experience in which he was discovering himself. The enemies had now become the children with whom he had to share the therapist.

In the next hour the nature of Dick's activity changed considerably. He had finished with the soldiers and animals. They had served their purpose in helping him to reach a point where he could be a little boy playing with an adult. He was fascinated with stamps and their value and rewrote his address. He told about his new school saying: "I know lots of kids there but at first I didn't know anyone and I was afraid." It was so clear that he was talking about his relation with the therapist that no interpretation was needed.

Again the medium of activity changed, and Dick decided to draw. The new content had, for a time, the same aggressive tone as the war play. But drawing was of his own creation while the soldiers were ready-made for him; thus this medium was an indicator of his movement toward facing more directly his own feeling. In the drawing he represented the therapist as "a funny looking guy," saying: "You have a stick and you're going to hit someone." At first Dick denied that he might be the object of this attack, or that he himself had any such impulses. A moment later his play, however, showed an acceptance that he was the one being chased. He made the therapist the big and dangerous person, and portrayed himself as strong enough to stand up against this force. Thus he first began to take back into himself some of the aggressiveness and power that he had projected, and had been able to own only in the objects of his identification. In his drawing he then showed how he was going to knock the therapist out.

There was an inevitable recoil from this rapid movement toward assertion and, after knocking the therapist out in the drawing, Dick pictured himself as in jail and being sent to the electric chair. Having punished himself for this bold assumption of power, he resumed, in his drawing, the aggressive role. "I'll sock this cop in the jaw. He is mad because I killed you and was ready to put me in the electric chair but I killed the cop." In this phantasy material he tested out the mounting feeling of himself in the therapeutic relation, and he gradually became a living person who was not overwhelmed either by his own aggressive impulses, for which he could now accept some responsibility, or by the power he projected on others who represented the potential threats to his uncertain feeling about himself. He was finding that he could live and use his strength in conjunction with the living qualities in others.

Dick terminated that hour by using various colors to indicate shades of feeling,[14] a medium he continued to use throughout most of his remaining hours. This first occurred as he accepted being a little angry when the therapist said his time was about up. He returned to his drawing, used some red paint and said: "This is where I jabbed you." He mentioned three colors in his drawing: "Blue is true. Red is to be bad," but changed that to "be brave." He put red on the figure that represented himself, adding: "Yellow, that means not brave." At the end of the hour he painted a blue cap on the figure of the therapist, which seemed to indicate his increasing feeling of confidence in this relationship which he was using to gain a sounder perception of his own strength.

In the next hour Dick brought a red apple and quickly announced: "We are both a little red today but we are also a little afraid." This was a particularly important step for this boy in whom feeling assumed such total proportions.

---

[14] Many children make fascinating and illuminating use of color in the therapeutic situation and an entire chapter might well be written on this subject.

When aggression is used to shut out fear it frequently becomes as complete as the fear, which can throw a child into
disorganized panic states. Dick began to find he could be
both aggressive and fearful, and this represented an important
growth step. With the coming of this more balanced attitude about himself he recalled his first hour and said: "You
remember when I first came I was worried. I was afraid I
wouldn't get home." When the therapist commented that
Dick didn't feel much red in himself then he smiled and
added, "No. I had a lot of yellow, didn't I?" The therapist,
in agreeing, emphasized how Dick was finding that he could
change those colors himself. He dropped the early defenses
he had built against getting into this relationship and spontaneously announced: "I will be glad to come next time. I
would be glad to come every day and keep those other kids
out, even if you were not here." [15]

In his eighth hour Dick started to paint and decided "not
to have any battle today." In a rather happy, confident mood
he brought up the problem of ending, saying: "How many
more times do I come?" Together we figured that he would
have five more appointments, a time that had to be set in part
by external circumstances and not solely by the movement
of the case.[16] With this more natural and adequate feeling
about himself, Dick's medium of expression again changed.
He wanted to hammer nails which, for him, was a more direct and constructively assertive expression of himself. This
roused uncertainty again, partly because he initiated the activity and partly because of the noise he made. Accordingly
he sought the therapist's support in this new activity. Dick

---

[15] The movement in this case up to this point shows the positive value
of resistance. Through resistance Dick had found his own strength, which
then he could use for his own development rather than against it as in
his fight against being influenced by anyone but himself. There is further
discussion of this in Chapter III.

[16] *See* Chapter IX for a more extensive discussion of this point.

introduced the change by saying: "I don't always have to paint." "Not unless you want to," he was told. "Do other boys hammer nails?" "Yes, and it sounds as if you would like it." But he had to protect himself from the dangers of this much freedom and added, "I might make too much noise." The therapist discussed the boy's determination not to take any chances. Dick insisted on his question: "Would you mind if I hammered?" and the therapist replied, "Dick, you seem afraid that I would. I guess you will just have to find out for yourself." It would have been easy but meaningless had the therapist been caught by Dick's fear at this stage and reassured him that it was all right. Dick was still using that fear to make the therapist assume the risks for him. Dick went ahead on his own initiative with the hammering and found, through his own medium of expression and through his own decision, what he actually could do. Only when the therapist would not take the responsibility of reassuring Dick, could he go ahead on his own.

Dick next explored another medium of expression and that too, like his previous ones, revealed the point at which he was in the precipitated growth experience which we call therapy. He wanted to take home what he was making, and tentatively and with uncertainty he made this request. For Dick the request had deep significance and was closely associated with his feeling about ending. It meant taking away and owning as his own a new self which he had built with the therapist's help. But guilt inevitably arose in him over his right to possess the new self which had emerged out of his relationship to the therapist. Here we see a universal growth dilemma: "Have I the right to be different from those who gave me life?" He dealt with that in this way: "If I made a toy could I give it to you?" When the therapist questioned: "Dick, do you really want to give it to me?" he took the next step, saying that he really wanted to take it home for himself. In this the therapist supported him. But this assertion of his own desire still aroused guilt. A moment later when a nail scratched the chair he condemned himself by saying: "I am bad." Again the therapist helped him by consenting that at times it was fun to be bad. Dick smilingly and easily accepted his right to some "badness" and went ahead to tell, "How pretty this toy will look in my room." Dick had now accepted his right to take something for himself without being inhibited by feeling guilty about asserting that right.

In the ninth hour Dick showed anxiety that was closely related both to ending and to his having gone so far ahead in his previous hour. He returned in an anxious mood to his painting activity, and used considerable yellow paint. The therapist helped him talk about some of the anger he had about having only four more visits and he timidly agreed, telling about a fight he had been in. "I hit him. I hit him so hard he fell into the street." I smiled and said that was quite a blow. Dick retracted a little, and said: "He stumbled," but added, "I took my part. I was brave that time."

It was fascinating to see how this boy used, as children frequently do, this outside experience of a fight to express his more immediate feeling. Dick was aware that that feeling belonged to the particular moment, and it was not necessary to talk about it. The therapist, sensing that Dick's anxiety about ending was contained in that remark, responded in a light tone that he would probably still be on his feet after the blow. Dick then wanted to borrow some of the therapist's courage and asked: "Do you feel a little brave?" From this the therapist and the boy agreed that it was possible to be brave even when one had, at the same moment, some of the fearful feelings. Dick ended the hour with a real assertion: "In that fight, I was all brave."

He was in a gay mood the next hour, and hid behind a

door in the waiting room when the therapist went for him. This was a daring act for him and took on significance far beyond the deed itself as it was associated with ending. It became a test of his bravery and he said: "That was a bad trick." But Dick was more intrigued now than worried with his "badness," and continued with his painting. He made the therapist a cowboy with a holster, saying: "You're going to hit me and I'm going to sock you in the nose." He drew and painted a picture portraying this action. By making the therapist the aggressor who instigated the conflict he allowed and justified a more aggressively alive feeling in himself. This was such a contrast to the timid and withdrawn little boy who, a few weeks earlier, could not initiate so much as a parade with the soldiers. While he still used the media of painting and play with the soldiers, he was now experiencing feelings that clearly belonged to him.

The next three therapeutic hours were full of animated activity, most of which had an assertive quality that still seemed somewhat alien to him. Dick was getting acquainted with the use of a quality in himself, in his relationship with the therapist which was now approaching an end. He was able to bring out quite clearly that he was ready to end but could also express the other side of his feeling when he said: "I don't feel like going." This was indication of his growth. He could be ready to go and feel regretful about taking that step. This was true likewise of his desire to be "bad." Dick's feelings now could be partial ones that allowed room for the existence of other feelings at the same time.

One more excerpt from Dick's last hours will round out the discussion of this case. Toward the end of the twelfth appointment he began a painting which he left unfinished saying: "I will finish this next time," which he knew would be his final hour. He made it clear that the figure he painted was the therapist, and he put gold trimming on the trousers.

In his last hour Dick started to finish the painting but first bragged about some mischief which he had been in at school. First he put his own name on the picture and wanted to be sure it would be placed "where other boys will know I did it. I am not taking this painting home." This decision had all the meaning of leaving a discarded part of himself with the therapist. He completed the picture and said of the therapist: "You have a sword and you are beating me with it. You are like a big giant. You ate more spinach than I did." The therapist commented: "You are leaving that dangerous man here." Dick agreed saying: "I will leave you all by yourself."

Then he added: "Now I will draw myself. I'm getting angry. I am going to be a bigger giant than you. I will be a millionaire giant. I have started to eat spinach myself. I am all red." It will be recalled that he had made red the symbol of bravery and danger. So he painted a large figure of himself in red, and put a little yellow on the figure of the therapist saying: "I'm all red, you have a little yellow on you." Then Dick completed the cycle by having the big "millionaire giant" overwhelm the other. He did this in a most friendly way, with no anxiety in it but with a comfortable sense of possession of his own power.

He followed this with a different painting which portrayed a house in which soldiers lived. Dick said: "You and I are friends, we are not fighting each other anymore. We have a little peace between you and me." When he found that he could own his own assertive feeling in relation to the power of another, he felt at peace. He had gained some perception of the value of his own separate self which was no longer in continuous jeopardy and which did not require of him either total submission or total assertion.[17]

---

[17] This boy needed much more help than it was possible to give in the limited time available. The anxiety he had in ending was greater than

This material was chosen with the primary purpose of showing the significance of shifting media of expression as a child progressed towards a fuller achievement of a self in the differentiating steps in the therapeutic relationship. In illustrating this much the case also revealed, in outline, the whole therapeutic process: the dynamics of the beginning phase; the interplay and shifting roles assigned by the boy to himself and the therapist as he differentiated himself in the steady framework which the therapist provided; and, finally, his readiness to end with the natural anxiety associated with accepting the ownership of a self built by his own participation in a relationship provided for him. The whole experience involved verbal and emotional content that stemmed from his relationship with the therapist. Little or no reference was made to his past or even to the current activities in his new home, where gradually he found a place for himself while therapy was going on.

An epitome of all that I have emphasized in this chapter about the value and meaning of the child's activity is contained in this material. Each shift in Dick's activity was understood and used for the meaning it had for this particular experience and at the moment of the child's perceiving this or that specific reaction. That these responses were rooted in his past deprivations can be accepted as true without, however, making it necessary to keep the boy endlessly shackled to those roots by the therapist's historical orientation to them. Dick's responses were used by the therapist

is found in children who are ready in themselves for it. Unfortunately he did not return in the fall as had been planned because the agency worker was reluctant to interrupt the fair adjustment he was making in his foster home. Two years later it was necessary for Dick to come to the clinic again and a longer period of treatment was possible at that time. On the whole we have found that children placed in foster homes and in institutions need a longer period of therapy than children who have parents who can share with the child an active part in therapy.

to call forth from this immediate experience the growth-inducing values that were implicit in it. What he did in play and the use he made of materials to objectify his changing roles provided sufficient verbal and feeling content.

6

A FEARFUL CHILD IN THERAPY
A CASE HISTORY

In this chapter, nineteen treatment interviews with a ten-year-old boy will be discussed in detail. Through this material, the therapeutic process can be studied as a continuing movement within the structure of a relationship that has a beginning, an intermediate phase, and an ending. Some of the material from the mother's interviews will also be included since the problem was closely interwoven with the mother's attitudes, and since her active participation was an important part of the progress of this case.

Reference has been made in an earlier chapter to the importance of the clinical structure as providing a setting for the growth-inducing experience which is therapy. That point is illuminated by the case material of this chapter. Mrs. Landis, mother of ten-year-old Solomon, had been taking him to various medical clinics for four years where he had been treated, on a symptomatic basis, for his tics and "nervousness." Altogether, ten doctors had taken part in his treatment which consisted of mild sedatives, tonics and reassurance of ultimate recovery. Both mother and boy were faithful and persistent in their visits.

Mrs. Landis, with some help from her medical advisers who finally recognized the emotional basis of her son's physical difficulties, began to want some different and more effective treatment. She saw the boy getting worse, and knew, in a vague way, that he was not being helped. When she was referred to the Child Guidance Clinic she had no idea what would be involved in this except that the treatment would be different. She came to the clinic with uncertainty and fear for her application interview. She told of her long period of worry over his tics which medicine had not helped, and said that she wanted and needed help.

In that first visit Mrs. Landis presented the problem in her boy, but what was more important, gained some understanding of what this new experience might be like for her. She learned that both she and Solomon would have regular weekly appointments, the boy with the psychiatrist and the mother with the social worker. There would be no medicine and probably no further physical examinations since these had been thoroughly and accurately done. In this new way of working the mother found she would be an active participant, not just the anxious mother who brought her son to be "cured" and who would wait in the reception room for him while that took place. She learned that the boy would have an opportunity to become acquainted with the doctor who would help him. He would have more to do than take medicine and listen to reassurances from the doctor. The mother, a simple but sensitive person, decided she wanted to get started, even though fearful of what this new experience might do to both of them. In making this decision the mother took an important step in giving up her adherence to a belief that Solomon's difficulties were caused by physical disorders.

Certain details concerning the background of this problem are important and bring out a fact I have mentioned before, that is a part of all emotional problems in children; the problem is not exclusively in the child nor in the parents but rather in their living relationship. These parents, of foreign background, had brought up their four children in this community. The oldest son, thirty and married, had achieved the success so ardently desired by the parents. He was the ideal son, serious, responsible and "leading the good life." The second son, twenty-two, was the antithesis of the first—irresponsible, shiftless, and dull. A sporadic attempt at marriage had failed and he returned home to live a parasitic existence. A daughter of seventeen presented no difficulties and was developing in a normal way.

Solomon came late in the parents' lives and was not wanted, a fact the mother was able to tell and discuss much later when she had acquired a healthier attitude about her relation to her boy.[1] Solomon was in a difficult spot in the family group as he carried the parents' hope that he would grow up to be like the first son and fear that he would be like the second. He had little chance just to be himself, which is the base on which healthy growth must rest. He was the object of anxious care and guidance, and the fact that he was described as a "very nervous child from birth" indicated the vicious cycle that had been established. The relationship of the parents, particularly the mother, to this boy rested on anxiety as to what he might become unless they did a great deal to insure his normal development. The mother's care was hovering and anxious and this may have had much to do with his being the "nervous child" she described him as being from infancy. The more nervous and fearful he became, the greater became the mother's apprehensiveness. Thus the incubating medium for Solomon's neurotic behavior pattern became more established

[1] An important principle in history taking is illustrated by this. Parents can bring out certain facts charged with their own emotional attitudes only at those points where these facts have a new meaning in terms of their own changes. It would have been meaningless to have tried to elicit this fact sooner. A good history is one that grows naturally out of the movement of the case.

The relationship between Solomon and his mother allowed little natural growth. The mother continued to give and give, but mainly in relation to Solomon's nervousness and increasing fear. The boy, in turn, was on the receiving end of the relationship and the more he received the more he demanded. Through the fears which led to his never going to bed alone and thus keeping the mother close to his side, he was warding off the achievement of any separateness or responsibility in himself. He clung to the undifferentiated relationship to his mother by his fears, and later by the tics which provided a somatic shield for the real fears Solomon had of any growth steps that might take him out of his cloistered existence. Mrs. Landis, in turn, held Solomon to her through her fear that he could not become adequate without her. She described his growing petulance and temper outbursts. These were usually precipitated by anything she did apart from him or when Solomon was held to some accountability for his own behavior.

Solomon was a bright boy and the one place he achieved success was in school. He did good school work but had few friends. Increasingly, he was regarded as "crazy Solomon" by the children in school and neighborhood.

This rough outline of the problem is enough to show that when the mother and boy came to the clinic together for their first appointment, they were bringing the real problem that lay in the undifferentiated nature of their relation. For this mother to let him have enough of his problem to come to the clinic himself and enter into a relationship with another person meant that she was taking a first step in finding a way of being his mother instead of the source of all his life force. For Solomon to leave his mother in the clinic waiting room and come with the therapist meant that he was risking the loss of his main life support without being sure he had anything in himself to take its place.

The following material shows the way in which the separate therapeutic interviews in the clinic gave significance to this new experience in terms of the whole problem between mother and son for which they needed help.

In the waiting room the mother and son sat close together. The social worker and therapist introduced themselves. As Solomon went with the therapist Mrs. Landis anxiously watched him leave. Then she went to the social worker's office. Parent and child had embarked on a new separation experience.

As he went into the therapist's office, Solomon smiled in a forced way. In appearance, he was pale, somewhat undernourished, and obviously fearful. There were a few facial tics. The therapist was friendly in a casual way as names were exchanged. Solomon made a feeble effort to cover the initial fear engendered by this new experience that separated him from his mother. For the moment he was cut adrift. He weakly said that the room looked cheerful enough but quickly got to his own anxiety and broke out into tears saying, "I'm just scared and I don't know what it is."

The natural, human reaction at this point would have been to reassure this frightened child by saying there was nothing to be afraid of, or that he would not be hurt. A responsible therapist, however, recognizes the importance of helping Solomon express his fear and come to terms with it. The therapist, on the other hand, who feels the necessity to relieve the child of his fear keeps the source of the relief in himself and so postpones the child's discovery of his own capacity to live through and to overcome his fear. In this instance, the therapist supported Solomon in his fear by saying that he knew how frightened he was of coming to this strange place, of going off with a strange man and leaving his mother outside. He was encouraged to talk about how he felt. At first Solomon was too choked up with tears to talk.

Soon he told of having gone to a hospital which made him worse and now he was afraid to take medicine. The therapist nodded and added that coming to the clinic had stirred the fear that this too would make him worse; maybe he thought that it had already made him worse because he had been so frightened. Solomon agreed and went on to tell how "the feeling starts in my foot," and he did not know exactly what he was afraid of. The therapist said: "Solomon, I know. You are afraid because you are in this room alone with a man you do not know and whom you cannot yet trust." A discussion followed about Solomon's coming regularly once a week and the therapist suggested that as they gradually became acquainted Solomon might get a better understanding of the fears he had.

At this point Solomon noticed a brief case in the office and asked, with suspicion and belligerence: "What's in that— what's behind it?" The casual comment was made that Solomon believed it held danger and maybe he would like to look for himself. He made his first move from the safe haven of his chair and investigated. The therapist asked what he expected to find and he said: "Maybe there is a gun." When he found nothing dangerous the therapist said: "You were able to find out for yourself, weren't you?" He agreed with a smile and for the first time in the interview, he was relaxed.

Fear, when it is this diffuse and has no content, is hard for any person to handle and may lead to panic. As the feeling becomes localized and a vehicle is found to mediate it, the intensity of the feeling diminishes. Solomon's first hour illustrated such a panic, with the diffusion of fear expressed in his comment: "I don't know what I am afraid of." He was helped to accept the fear as belonging to the immediate experience. Then he was able to project the cause of the feeling on the brief case. As he examined this the fear was lessened since he himself had done something about his fear.

This, however, was the reverse of most of his previous life experiences where, on the basis of having fear, he could make everyone else do something about it. The control held in the fear reaction is tremendous, and Solomon found in it his most effective weapon for shielding himself from the demands of growth.

In the first fifteen minutes of this initial therapeutic interview a pattern for later reactions was established. Solomon came in a panic, but after fifteen minutes he was relaxed. Such a transformation must have seemed like magic. Thus arose an impression of which he made much more later: that the therapist possessed a magic power that would cure his fears and tics without requiring anything of him. In stressing this he tried to maintain his old pattern of living, through another person's strength, a reaction that could be expected at this point. However, he also found in this first hour that he held the cure of his fears in himself and that the doctor, instead of being the cure, was the supporter and clarifier of his own efforts.

In the latter half of that treatment hour Solomon was much freer. He described his feeling of fear as going away, and agreed to the comment: "You found you could be afraid and could do something about it yourself." He proceeded to tell more of his fears and of his efforts to sleep alone. "I did sleep alone for three nights. I couldn't believe it was me who did that." He went on, with more determination than fear, to tell how he makes his mother sleep in the room with him because "I am afraid."

In the last few minutes of that hour, when he was quite at ease, Solomon allowed himself to start playing with the toy soldiers. In the aggressive phantasy of his play a sick girl on the way to a hospital was being attacked by German soldiers who wanted to kill her. As the time was up this could go no further, but it seemed to crystallize the same fear that had been aroused in him when he was brought to the clinic, which for him was just the same as a hospital. As he was leaving he volunteered that he had been frightened but could agree, with some relief, when the therapist repeated: "Yes, and you did something about it."

This first interview with this neurotic ten-year-old boy clarified a number of points, both in the boy's presentation of the problem and in the form this problem took in the therapeutic hour. The absorbing nature of the mother-son relationship was revealed by the amount of fear that was roused in their brief separation. Just coming into the office without the maternal support brought Solomon's essential problem into the foreground and gave the therapeutic situation an immediate connection with his emotional disturbance. Mother and son hardly existed as separate individuals, but were fused into an undifferentiated whole held together by the mother's seeing Solomon as a sick boy who needed all that she was trying to give and by his maintaining the role of a sick child by the determined and persistent use of fears and "nervousness." Here is the vicious cycle in which the mother gives so much to make the child well and the child continues to require that support by staying sick and making others assume the responsibility for curing him.

Considerable space could be devoted to the historical development of the case but that is not the major focus of this discussion. The mother had a neurotic orientation to this boy, her youngest and last child. Pride in creation and guilt of failure met in her feeling about the boy and bound him to her in a way that allowed little growth. She could not take chances and the boy, sensing his power, held her to him by his neurotic symptoms.

Whatever the cause of the problem, this mother and son nevertheless wanted a different relationship to each other. That was the motive behind their seeking the clinic's help.

The therapeutic problem now became one of helping them to find a new orientation to the reality of their own separate but related selves. The mother really was tired of carrying the load for her son, yet she was caught by her own fear of what would happen if she gave a sharper definition to her own mother role. Her description of Solomon as a nervous child from birth grew from the fear that he could not be altogether responsible for the self she had created.

The therapeutic problem now became clearer. Could this mother and child be helped to break up their self-destroying closeness and find a new way to live together? How could they be supported and helped to live through the struggle for and against this movement toward self-realization? How could this boy use the therapist to gain a different sense of responsibility for himself, without getting caught in another binding relationship? How could the therapist give help without becoming the cure which would allow the boy to disown any sense of participation in his own growth? These are questions that arise in one way or another in every therapeutic experience and some light may be thrown on them by a consideration of Solomon's progress.

Several other points should be re-emphasized here before we proceed with the boy's material. Solomon and his mother came together and participated in this new venture since the problem was in their relationship. She took the initiative in this experience, whereas Solomon was brought to the clinic with the implication that he was to be changed. Even though he was outwardly willing to be brought, he felt, as an attack on him, the fact that his whole way of living was exposed to the possibility of being changed by this new person. He had had considerable experience, during four years of medical treatment, of warding off the curative efforts of others. The fear in this first hour was partly the fear engendered by separation from his mother. But the fear was also closely related to the possible power of the therapist to change him, the fear of having his "fears" taken away. The phantasy of being attacked and killed, which came out at the end of the hour, was significant of this boy's feeling about the therapist's power to change him.

The hour itself defined another dilemma. Solomon tried to project all of the curative responsibility on to the therapist. In this way he sought to avoid any self-responsibility for change, and to remain free to struggle against being changed. But in the first hour a "miracle" happened. He came in with great fear and then he had the unique experience of being helped to express the fear and so to modify his own feeling. There was momentary relief in this. But he used this to invest the therapist with magical powers to cure him, retaining for himself again the passive role he had played for years, a role invested with his counterpower to ward off change. By assuming weakness and an inability to do anything himself he had in reality been stronger than anyone else. But it was a strength that could not be used creatively. It could only be used negatively. When Solomon said in a later hour, "I have come to be cured," he was trying to perpetuate the magic effect of that first hour to avoid any further risking of his own participation, which could lead to self-definition.

In the second treatment hour, a week later, Solomon was more at ease and commented: "The room looks different." The therapist agreed that it might look different because he was feeling different. Solomon overlooked that and went ahead, finding in the new arrangement of chairs and toys a vehicle to explain some of his own feeling of change.[2] In the first hour he tried to find in the room the cheerfulness he could not feel in himself, and in this second hour he

[2] This illustrates the value of having interviews in the same room—a point that is stressed in Chapter IV.

again attributed the change to the room. He had so little feeling of himself as a separate entity that he could not trust any values that had meaning in terms of himself. Of that second hour, he said that he had wanted to come and was "excited and nervous but I am more used to it."

Solomon's activity reflected the disorganized quality in himself. He made sporadic efforts to play but in this there was no continuity. He was torn between the desire to use play to isolate himself from the strange new influence of the therapist, and the intriguing desire to do more with him. It was with relief that he discovered the checkerboard which allowed joint activity in a game he knew. But he carefully avoided taking any credit for his knowledge and said: "I can play because my brother taught me and he is the neighborhood champion." He referred here to the brother who had been such a failure.[3] He could play but one game for he was anxious to get to "more important things." His distrust of the new experience appeared in his statement about a "psychologist who came to help my brother and he said he would come and help me—but he fooled me, he didn't come. The man said if I came nine times I would get well. I went eight times. My mother was in the room when I went to see him. He was the angry type." This statement was referred to his relationship here, to what he had expected, and to the dangers involved in his being alone with the therapist. He could agree to this saying: "Yes, I guess I was wrong."

Solomon was troubled and puzzled about his mother's participation in the clinic experience, as shown in his comments: "My mother does not know what this room is like," "she sits in the waiting room," and, "she wants me to come alone." At this point it would have been less puzzling but also less therapeutic if he had come alone to the clinic. In that way he could have kept his experience at the clinic from

[3]This fact will be discussed later in the case.

touching the intrenched position he held at home through the persistent use of his fears and the maintenance of the facial tics. But when he and the mother had equal but separate parts in seeking help, that isolation could not be maintained. They had the opportunity to break up the old and to find, at the same time, a new balance in their relationship. Naturally, it was baffling; even more, it stirred anxiety. Solomon knew that his mother did not sit in the waiting room but he wanted to maintain that illusion. He had to face the fact, with me in this hour, that his mother was taking an active part, too. This was his own first move toward becoming a person in his own right.

In these first two hours a great deal happened. Solomon experienced a surge of feeling, and through that he became quickly engaged in this new relationship. The tone and movement of the following hours stemmed from this beginning. At the end of the second hour he commented on "the short time," and added, "I wish I could stay two hours." While there was relief in this comment it was also the beginning of his struggle to control the direction of this new experience. We will soon see how much reliance he placed on time to effect a change, on the hope that all he had to do was to present himself in the clinic in order that the "magic" could do its work.

Solomon's previous experience provided some basis for this fight since he had accepted no part in the creation of his fears and therefore could place all of the curative efforts outside himself. This pattern had been reinforced by the four years of medical treatment. When he started this new and, for him, unique experience, he became panicky and then found immediate relief. Truly there was magic in this new place and he could justify his belief that all he had to do was to come to the clinic and the cure would follow. But out of this very dilemma sprang the opportunity for the therapist to give direction to the therapy. Solomon, in struggling to maintain his nonparticipating role, became through these efforts an active partner in the process of change. He had to participate most actively in order to keep from participating in this experience! Herein are the positive and therapeutic values of resistance. But it took clear and direct definition on the part of the therapist for Solomon to make constructive use of this negative effort.

I have mentioned the relief which accompanies the sudden and, at times, dramatic change frequently occurring in the beginning hours of treatment. There is, however, another side to this phenomenon. Anxiety is often stirred by the power of this experience which gives some children, as well as adults, the feeling of having but little self if they can "be changed" so mysteriously. They are left feeling so vulnerable. But the defense against being changed, sometimes misunderstood as resistance, helps the patient to regain a feeling of himself, particularly if the therapist has not assumed the role of healer through the purposeful application of his own power.

Coming to the clinic was still "exciting" to Solomon as the third hour began, but "the room has not changed this week." He was more defensive and evasive in expressing any feeling. He started with: "My mother thought I wasn't coming," but disowned this idea as originating with himself. He wanted to play checkers, and did so indifferently. He was having greater difficulty in finding an external medium to carry his feeling of change, and he said: "My mother thinks I am better," and spoke of "being tired of seeing the same old things." The therapist said that the way Solomon feels and not the way the old or new toys look is the important consideration. He talked, then, more about his fears. He was startled when the therapist commented on the usefulness of his fears in controlling so much of his life. To this remark, which was a little too much for him at this point, he responded by repeating: "You get tired of seeing the same old things."

It was interesting that the mother described little change at this time but emphasized instead, how bad his tics had been. She was clinging to her old conception of Solomon as sick. Mrs. Landis also talked about his interest in doing more things and described how lonely she felt. Her remark, "What will I have left when the children are grown," summed up her great feeling of loss in the growth of her sons. There was the fear that when Solomon took on more responsibility for himself, she would be left with no one needing her.

The facial tic was an obsessive motor act that, curiously enough, was absent during most of his therapeutic hours. During this early period it was most prominent at home. A theoretical explanation of this fact lies in the use of this persistent motor equivalent of anxiety as an effective shield for feeling.

In his relation to the therapist Solomon's determined and almost obsessive need to make the therapist his cure was the equivalent of the motor tic. Moreover it served somewhat the same purpose; that is, protection against the feeling aroused by any move toward self-definition and self-responsibility. As long as he could sit back, as he did for several weeks, and bask in the belief that the doctor and time would bring about the "desired" cure, he had little anxiety. At home the facial tic had become, concurrently with the persistent and obsessive use of the idea of fear, the symbol of his being sick and in need of all the mother continued to give. Thus he was protected by everyone's acceptance of him as a sick boy.

But in his therapeutic hours he was singularly free of the facial tics. The explanation of this seems clear. In the first therapeutic hour Solomon was precipitated into a relationship that involved real feeling on his part. The fears he had been talking about and using became real. But the movement away from fear, through the awakening of a sense of his own capacity to handle it, renewed his struggle to avoid the waking up process which is growth. There, in that first hour, began the projection of the cure on the therapist, and an attempt to evade his own part in it. This evasion carried, as I have said, the same obsessive force that maintained the tic. But there was an essential difference: the tic protected him from any real relationship between himself and anyone else. This new expression of feeling brought him into an actively dynamic relationship with the therapist.

A tic, or any other hysterical conversion phenomenon, not only serves as a somatic shield against feeling; in doing that it also serves as an insulation against any real relationship with others. Through this symptom an individual establishes a one-way traffic basis; he can get from others what he needs and give nothing in return. Solomon got everything from his mother and gave nothing. He was able to maintain that same position with the ten doctors in whose defeat he gloried. He tried to maintain the same pattern in this therapeutic experience, and it was the growing intensity of these efforts that broke down the insulating devices. A real boy began to emerge.

The therapeutic difficulty encountered with children having tics, particularly speech tics, centers around the isolation they can maintain with a therapist. The somatic barrier that disguises real feelings is an effective one and "the grand indifference" of the hysteric is common with them. The result is that effective therapeutic connection is difficult to make with such a child or adult. Solomon might have established himself on this more isolated basis, had his protection against his anxiety held in that first hour.

As he came to the office for his fourth hour, Solomon kept on his hat and coat. No words could describe more clearly the guarded quality there was in him. He went directly to the checkerboard saying: "I like this best." The game had provided a safety spot and in that sense the play was valuable. But the fact that he was clinging to that evasion required some direct handling by the therapist, who commented: "You feel more confidence when you have this game, and evidently you are determined that nothing different shall happen." He agreed and pointing to the toys added: "I'm not used to them yet." There still was necessity in going along slowly with him as he reached out cautiously to anything new.

The meaning and the use of play in therapy has been more fully discussed in Chapter V. But it can be re-emphasized here that the particular type of play activity chosen frequently is the indicator of where the child is in his therapeutic experience. When a child changes, it is reflected in the shifting character of the play; if he does not change, then the struggle will focus in this determination to do one thing and only one thing. It is the use a child makes of play and not the particular thing with which he plays that has significance.

Toward the end of the hour, a time when children frequently find it safer to experiment, Solomon left the checkers and played with the animals. They again provided an external medium for measuring his own growing sense of difference, and it meant a good deal when he said: "These are different from the ones I have at home." What he really meant was that he was beginning to feel a little different from the way he did at home, and while he was intrigued with his own change he was anxious about it at the same time. This was discussed quite simply and in terms of his growing freedom to do more than to play checkers. He seemed to understand this and added: "I am getting acquainted." Then he became braver and entered upon a few minutes of more aggressive play with the soldiers and guns, and as the hour ended he said: "Next time I might want to start playing with them right away." He agreed with me that we could wait and see how he felt next time.

A week later Solomon took off his coat and started at once to play with the soldiers. The fact that he was free to play in this new medium made it less necessary for him to play [4] and soon he was talking about his "sickness." He was more accepting of a new feeling in himself when he said: "Two years ago I was told I would get better when I was older, and now I am older." The therapist entered this discussion and commented on how he had felt then, that his part had been to sit back and to wait for time to pass; but that he was beginning to find that growing up was not something to put off but that he could take a real part in it. The boy was active in this discussion and talked more about how he had been placed in hospitals with everyone telling him that he was sick. The therapist agreed that it was not easy to give up that idea, particularly since now he had started to give it up. Solomon assented, "Yes, I'm nervous. I can't exercise." The therapist wanted to know what was stopping him and he asserted: "The doctor said not to, and when I came here I thought this would be a hospital and I would get medicine." This was not entirely a complaint but partly an acceptance of the difference between the old and new way of getting help. Solomon had begun to feel the meaning of what he was doing. Naturally, ambivalent feelings arose; one of relief over his improvement, but the other a determination to test out his capacity to prevent this new experience from being different from the old. The feeling of relief became

---

[4] By this I mean that play, particularly for older children, is an indirect therapeutic medium of expressing ideas and feelings.

more prominent as the interviews continued. He was now changing within the safe confines of his relationship with a therapist who could share some of the responsibility of helping this to happen. This gave his change more meaning because he was achieving it with the help of another and not just through his own isolated effort.

In telling about his sleeping habits, Solomon explained how he had stopped sleeping alone after hearing someone talk about dying; this caused him to worry about his mother's dying, and he described his need to watch her closely. The prominent anxiety feature of children who present this dependent picture springs from the lack of differentiation between themselves and the parent. The adult represents so much of the child's life force that any move which breaks up this relationship, such as the separation at night, starting school, or an experience such as therapy, may seem like death to the child. For Solomon these separation requirements aroused the death fear but now he could talk about his fear aroused in the therapeutic experience because of the steps he had taken toward some acceptance of his new ability to maintain life through the use of his own capacities.

Solomon continued to do a great deal in his fifth interview and seemed to be taking hold of a new quality in himself when he described the advantage of being little (which he placed at three) and the difficulties of being big (which he placed at ten). In this therapeutic hour he made it clear that he did not want to wait until "I am big before I get well. If I get well when I am big it might come back." Getting big and getting well were synonymous with him and both had represented great danger. But he was intrigued with the progress he was making, and volunteered, "Maybe I can start going to bed by myself. I did it for three nights once." He blamed an external influence, the movies, for his backsliding but concluded: "The night will come, so I guess I have to see what I can do about it."

It was in this period that Solomon was telling his parents that his doctor wanted him to go upstairs alone. In doing this he was using his therapist as the initiator of a step which involved yielding to his maturing desires. Solomon was freer to use the therapist in this way because there had been no pressure in his therapeutic hour for this or any other particular type of change. He was not yielding to the overt desires of the therapist but was using him to support and justify his own readiness to yield on this important point. Solomon's refusal to go to bed alone had been one of his chief weapons in his control of his mother—in fact the whole family.

For a therapist to introduce into this relationship desires and pressures to bring about particular shift in behavior either precipitates a negative struggle against doing what the therapist wants him to do or a passive acceptance of the change asked. In the first instance the patient is blocked in arriving at his own readiness to do something different, and in the second instance he can divorce himself from the responsibility for what happens. In either instance no move would have been made by the individual to gain a sense of ownership and responsibility for the change he brings about. In this case the therapist could casually encourage Solomon to go ahead with his announced plan to change his sleeping habits. But it had to be casual, otherwise Solomon would have been quick to sense the therapist's eagerness for him to do this and ascribe the whole idea to him. In this way Solomon could, as he had been able to do so frequently, disown his own plan of action and say, in effect, "I did what you wanted. I tried to sleep alone and couldn't." What he actually did was to make the external act of going to bed alone proof of doing his part but nothing more.

This became clearer in the next two hours when he made an interesting use of this external change. In the sixth hour he reported on his success in sleeping alone when he first arrived and then settled into a detached type of play which took no apparent direction. In the seventh hour he told, in an overanxious way, of more improvement. "I could do more if my father didn't go upstairs ahead of me. If he goes up first it doesn't count." He went on to tell how he insisted that no one go upstairs ahead of him and found in this new sleeping plan some of the old control he exercised over the family when he insisted one of them accompany him to bed.

The therapist introduced a discussion of what these interviews meant to Solomon and of how he felt about them. The boy spoke, in the person of his brother, about his feeling and reported the brother as saying: "Why do you waste your time going there." He himself denied vigorously any ownership of such thoughts but went on to say: "I don't know how to get well just by coming here—but I have six months." A discussion followed which brought Solomon closer to the struggle he was putting into what he termed "getting well," and he clearly described the "cure" as what was done to him while his role remained passive. Again he spoke of his previous experiences with doctors and nurses. "When I went to see them, all I had to do was just what they told me." He was rebelling hard against any sense of his own participation. But it was through his fight to maintain the passive position that he took a much more active role. As previously stated, it is in such material as this that we gain a clearer picture of the value of resistance.

The therapist's role was not an easy one. This form of passive struggle which followed the formula "I'll do anything you want" is a difficult type of struggle to deal with. The child who can say openly, "I don't want anything from you; I will get well in my own time," usually is more ready to take help. The parasitic nature of this boy's problem and his pattern of living made it hard for him to be more direct. The therapeutic task was, therefore, to help him bring his feelings more into the open. In order to accelerate that, two points had to be kept clear; one, the nature of what the boy was doing in therapy and the feeling that was aroused; two, the therapist's maintaining a role with him that allowed the projection of the curing force without, however, accepting it and trying to make that projection come true through the therapist's desires and efforts. Solomon had been caught in that type of relationship with his doctors for years because they had allowed little opportunity for him to gain any feeling of his own participation in "getting well." All he had to do with them was to go faithfully, take their medicine and remain sick. In not taking over the responsibility for curing, the therapist was not playing a trick or even applying a "technique." He was giving reality to a conviction that there can be no change or cure except that which stems from the individual's readiness to be different. So, in this hour, Solomon was told that the therapist was not concerned with whether he went to bed alone or not; he was concerned, however, with Solomon's feeling of readiness to be more grown-up, the evidence of which might be shown in the change in his sleeping habits. He was told if he went to bed alone it would be because he felt ready to do so, and not because the therapist required it. He was quite sober and verbally took little part in this discussion.

The same pattern continued into the next hour. With a tense and unhappy look Solomon told of going to bed alone six times—"more than ever." He was encouraged in these efforts by friendly comments about his successes. He went on to say, "If other boys can do it, I can." His reporting job was over in the first ten minutes and then he settled into a corner and fussed with the toys. There was little purpose or continuity in his activity. He maintained this isolated position until a comment was made about how he was keeping his feelings to himself and shutting out the therapist. This brought a blast of feeling. "This play makes me sick." The therapist agreed that he probably felt that way about his aimless play and also felt that way about his weekly visits. The boy had been shooting with a toy cannon and added, "I mean shooting and missing all the time makes me sick." The therapist added, "You don't mean sick, Solomon, you mean that it makes you mad but it is hard for you to admit such feelings here." He agreed. This discussion resulted in the wider scattering of his effort and further isolation from the therapist.

Finally the therapist asked: "Solomon, what are you doing?" "I am trying to do everything," he replied and he continued in his scattered activity. A direct discussion of his determination to do nothing beyond merely keeping his weekly appointments brought an evasive response. "When I come to see you I don't think—when I don't think of things I don't get afraid." His coming was discussed as requiring some thinking activity and to this he agreed and added, "I have to get well. I have to get well myself." There was discussion of how he swung from the extreme of putting the whole job on the doctor to trying to do the whole thing himself, and his persistent response was: "I just think coming here will get me well." He was clinging desperately to the pattern of expecting everything by doing nothing but at the same time he seemed to sense the value of what he was doing with the therapist.

A person like this who fights to make another responsible for all change (and this happens commonly with both adults and children) must have a therapist who can define and maintain his therapeutic role if there is to be any progress. To the patient this may seem like a stubborn refusal to assume the responsibility inherent in the concept of "doctor," and that may lead to the type of deadlock described in Chapter VIII. But the therapist can define his own role in this relationship by recognizing and respecting the importance of the patient's struggle. He must know that the patient cannot get any help in a vacuum nor in a cold unresponsive medium. The therapist must bring to this relationship a human warmth and friendliness which does not engulf the child nor prevent a direct and sharp handling of the type of determination revealed by this boy. Actually Solomon had no experience in a relationship that allowed giving and taking. He was like a sponge, taking up much but giving back little. The struggles that have been described in therapy to this point were an essential part of his learning to live the role of Solomon in a relationship with one who did not relieve him of the need and opportunity to be himself. Only in this way could he differentiate his own strength from that of the therapist. It was this that he was doing. The therapist was not trying to break down his resistance but was refusing to be his cure and to take over the responsibility that Solomon was thrusting upon him.

The ninth hour was a climactic interview which brought to a focus all that had gone into the preceding weeks. Solomon looked languid and worried, but maintained his customary rigorous control of feeling. The therapist commented on his worried appearance but he was evasive and withdrew into a corner with a few toys. When this need to escape was mentioned, he shrugged his shoulders saying, "I just know I come here." Knowing how important it was for him to face and experience the pain of this immediate reality, if he were to move beyond this protective barrier, the therapist again opened the discussion of what he was doing and how he was feeling about coming. "I think there is nothing to it—it doesn't make sense." The therapist agreed with this if Solomon had to continue putting the whole job of getting well on the doctor. With more anxiety he said: "I don't know how to get well." At this point the therapist reversed the emphasis and said: "The harder job is being well and you are frightened now because you are closer to being well." It was true that this new responsibility he was taking for himself meant a breaking up of the dependent bond to his mother, which he had maintained through sickness. Each step he made away from sickness meant a step toward a more mature relationship with the mother; it also meant establishing his relationship with his therapist on the basis of getting well and not by remaining "sick."

As Solomon withdrew into solitary play the therapist discussed the tenacious way in which he clung to the idea of sickness. To be sick was to be safe as long as others would do the worrying. He almost agreed with this, and the therapist then commented on how he was finding this experience different in that it gave *him* a chance to do part of the job, not just to take a bottle of medicine. "That didn't do any good," Solomon said. The therapist agreed and added that Solomon was frightened at the moment because "this was doing him some good." The mother reported a great deal of change in her son but added that his tics were as bad as ever. Through these difficult therapeutic hours very few tics were noticeable.

Solomon was silent after this, and the therapist withdrew saying that he was there to help him further when he was ready for it. The directness of this discussion had pushed Solomon momentarily further into his shell. But his play had more purpose and much more feeling and he made a vehement attack on the soldiers. The therapist commented on "those soldiers getting a real punishing" and added that probably some of that anger was meant for him. That touched off the explosion and the barrier he had established to hold back his feeling melted. In angry crying he blurted: "I would rather be like I was than go through this." He summed up so much in this statement, and showed how aware he was of change in himself and of the amount of anxiety that was stirred by his movement away from his tight and undifferentiated way of living. His anxiety was now concerned with a new responsibility for himself which sprang directly from his growing relationship with the therapist. As the boy continued his angry outbursts of "What's the use of all this" the therapist was very gentle in his support. Then suddenly, in a tone that was more grieved than angry Solomon remarked: "You said you didn't care whether I went to bed alone or not." This had happened in an earlier interview when he was trying to prove that by going to bed alone he was doing what the therapist wanted him to do. He was trying at that time to avoid any self-initiated responsibility in that change. The therapist replied: "You are quite right, Solomon. I said that and meant it. I also said I did care about what you wanted and were ready to do about that—so if you are going to bed alone it is because you are ready and want to do it." He nodded agreement but maintained this struggle against his part in the changes that had been occurring. He repeated: "I'd rather be the way I was. People told me coming here would make me well." The fact that he was finding some truth in this but not on the pattern he had planned activated a more significant anxiety that emerged from his change. No doubt he was baffled, as anyone would be, who, in fighting against change, found he was participating in bringing it about.

The force Solomon had put into these interviews was clearly revealed toward the end of this dramatic hour. Again he said he didn't know how to get well, and we discussed the more important and harder task of knowing how to *be* well. Following this he said: "What do I have here that I don't have at home?" The therapist said: "Your relation with me." For a boy who had no attachment to anyone but his mother, this was too much and he let go with a final blast of his determination: "I will always be sick, nothing can make me well." In effect, he was trying to deny his growing relationship with the therapist and to assert his desire to recapture the safer and undifferentiated relationship with the mother from which both he and his mother were moving away. His divided feeling about being well was discussed and it was brought out that he was ready for something different but that he had to fight against that readiness at the same time.

Solomon really suffered in this hour. He was cringing in a corner and hardly moved an inch, but he could share his anger and fear and it had real meaning to him when, at the end of the hour, the therapist said: "Solomon, I think you and I are beginning to get somewhere."

In the following hour this boy came to the clinic for the first time without his mother. She could not let him come alone and sent the brother with him. Actually, Solomon brought the brother and told the therapist how he had to show him the way to the clinic. While he was quite tense, he was much less withdrawn, and even as he said, "I know I have to cure myself," he was giving the therapist a real part in this. He spoke of going to bed by himself and said: "I keep you in mind as I do it." He was accepting more support in his progress. It was disturbing to come without his mother as evidenced in his comment, "When my mother comes, the nurse tells her all that happened." Thus he maintained a necessary connection between his relationship to his therapist and the mother. But coming without the mother sharpened the meaning of his relationship to the therapist and he could now bear it.

The twelfth hour marked a real change in Solomon. Here was the beginning of a new and important ending phase of therapy. Solomon was freer, complained of the gap made necessary by a holiday and said: "Two weeks is too long to wait." Again he noticed new things in the office, talked about school and how much he liked it. Then he wanted to play a game of checkers. There was a different use of checkers than in previous hours. Earlier he had clung to that as the one safe and familiar spot; now he was playing a game with the therapist. He played a good game and he commented that it was the best he had played. At the end of the hour he went to the blackboard and wrote his name in Hebrew. This was a symbol not only of the increasing ownership of himself but also of his difference from the therapist. It was a meaningful and significant act and needed no interpretation.

Through the period covered by these crucial interviews, the mother was becoming more and more at ease with the boy. She was delighted with his progress, not only in his sleeping habits, but in the fewer temper outbursts and in his more mature behavior. Solomon could even let visitors come to the house without creating a disturbance to draw the mother back to him. Previously, that had been one of his favorite tricks. She was becoming the mother to this boy and not merely the continuous source of meeting all of his needs. She talked about the strange but good feeling of being through with doctors and went back over the long and fruitless search for help which only made the problem worse. She could talk about the difficulties presented by the other son without drawing Solomon into these. To her, he was becoming a boy and not just the symbol of the hope or the fear he long had been. In her own change she was really supporting the boy in his growth, and Solomon's interviews showed how much he needed her in this new role.

After a week's break Solomon was rather quiet. "I thought I might not get up in time." The therapist suggested that he felt less need of coming but he had to deny the ending impulse in this statement. He talked about a concert he had attended and complained about the adults who sat at the table for refreshments and "the kids could not." The therapist said: "Kids do have a hard time as the grownups seem to get the best of it." He agreed with vigor and could not see many advantages in being a "kid"; "I want to grow up." This carried the new orientation he was gaining about himself.

He brought out some interesting material when the subject of dreams came up. First he said, "I never dream," but then told of a dream when he was standing on the roof. "My mother tells me that dreams mean that God will make me live longer." He still had to make God and his mother responsible for his life force. He went on to say, "I dream of angels and my sister dreams about fire." He was puzzled because "My sister is not scared of going upstairs but I am." The therapist commented that he reserved all the pleasant things for his dreams and had all his fears when awake and his sister did the reverse. He agreed and went on to say, "I am still scared to go up without the lights. In the daytime I am not scared and then I think how crazy it is to be scared at night. I think I will practice without the light."

Solomon was much freer in talking about his "fears" and seemed to have much less fear of being afraid. He was more confident as he went on to compare the advantages of bigness and littleness and could see values in both: "Before, I didn't want to grow up—now I do." He was not too sure of this but was testing out the two sides of his feeling. He still insisted on describing the new in himself in external terms. When a comment was made about this he said: "I have been living in the same house for a long, long time," and agreed that it was hard to move out. "I am sick of it—I stay in the house—some people don't like to get big because they think they will have to work, but I want to get big—at least I want to see what it feels like." Actually, he was doing this within the framework of his therapeutic relationship. He talked in glowing terms about his oldest brother and how he wanted to live with him because "there are fewer opportunities to be scared." He was using his older brother to symbolize this new and growing feeling of being well; he was also testing out his readiness to end his interviews with the therapist.

In the beginning hours of therapy Solomon's primary identification was with his "sick" brother. It was this brother who had taught him checkers because "he is the best player in the neighborhood." This brother likewise was used by Solomon to support his feeling that no one could help him, and that it was a waste of time and money to try. When he was clinging tenaciously to his "sick" self he was caught between his fear of becoming like this brother and his need to use the brother to justify his own infantile pattern of behavior. Children always need their identifications with others, particularly with parents and siblings, to give completeness to their own growing but incomplete sense of self. They will use these identifications in building their relationship with a therapist, or, as frequently happens, to avoid getting into a relationship. Solomon had struggled hard against having anything but a passive relationship with his therapist. The first effect of therapy therefore was to bring out and to accentuate his use of these parasitic identifications. Thus, he was enabled to move away from them through establishing a relationship with the therapist which permitted a more mature feeling about himself to emerge. The oldest brother, who represented to Solomon strength and being well, now had a new and significant meaning for him. He felt an increasing identification with that brother as this came to have greater reality in terms of his own development.

One thing that stood out in this case was the insignificant and ineffectual role of the father. In many cases in which the problem is centered in an undifferentiated mother-son relationship, the movement in therapy brings the father into a different and more important relationship with the child. The child frequently talks more about the father and begins to imitate him in manner and deed. In this case the father apparently had little effective place in the presence of such a powerful maternal force. In an early interview the mother, in speaking of her husband, said: "He worries about this boy, but he is a man and leaves most of it up to me." At least she took the responsibility on her own shoulders. For Solomon the older son really represented the father role. There was twenty years difference in their ages so that it was natural for Solomon to find in his older brother the identification he needed as framework for his growing self.

Solomon's use of the older brother in his therapeutic hours was his first clear step towards ending his interviews with the therapist. Ending is the final phase of differentiation between therapist and child. The child's new feeling about himself finds expression, in feeling and content, in terms of his outside and continuing reality. Solomon was doing that as he talked about his brother, emphasizing how he liked him and how he wanted to live in his home.

In the thirteenth hour Solomon mentioned his tics for the first time. He introduced the subject by saying that his back hurt from twisting his neck around. He told of seeing a boy doing that and of how he found himself imitating him but "I really can't help doing it." The therapist responded, "And I suppose you still want me to say you can't." He nodded, saying, "The other doctors said I couldn't help it." The therapist commented: "Solomon, you were quite active in taking on that habit so I guess you can do something about dropping it." This puzzled him, since he doubted his ability to do that. Again the therapist defined his role by remarking: "All right, if you are that helpless about it, I suppose you will have to keep that habit." Then they talked more about the strength of his determination of which he still made use to hold others responsible for changing him. He had not given up that struggle, in fact the move toward ending had probably intensified it temporarily.

The emphasis that Solomon placed on the physical pain associated with his muscular contortions was a new factor which may have been his way to explain the fact he had fewer tics. When the pain ceased he could then say he felt better and thus justify the disappearance of the tics. Actually the tics were less noticeable after this. A similar sequence was clearly brought out by a seven-year-old girl who had a remarkable gait disturbance, characterized by contortions of the back and stiffness of the left leg.[5] For months she had crawled around the house and neighborhood and in her first therapeutic hour whirled rather than walked into the office. Three weeks later she complained for the first time of a severe pain in her back. The following day she announced: "My back does not hurt," and went out and played ball with her brothers. That was the beginning of a more normal gait which in six months became completely natural.

In the fourteenth hour, Solomon continued to emphasize that he came to be cured and "there is nothing to do here." In this hour he took less initiative, and the therapist commented that he seemed to be about through coming to the clinic. His reaction to this was interesting. He tried to end his therapeutic experience by making it appear that he had

[5] In this case I was indebted to Dr. Louis Casamajor of New York for the thorough neurological examination which established the hysterical nature of this child's unusual gait disturbance.

never really begun it, saying: "I did not want to come in the first place"; then added, "Sometimes I don't want to come, there is never anything to do here." But in these efforts to deny the meaning of his therapeutic relationship in order to dilute or to evade facing how much it meant, he actually was much more related to the therapist. There was none of his former cringing in the corner, and the tone of his talking was not against but far more with his therapist. He was in a more reflective mood as he said: "Sometimes I just want to wait for getting well. They say you get well anyway when you are older and sometimes I believe these habits will go away without my doing anything about them."

Although the words sounded like his old fight to shift the responsibility and to use "the doctors" to support his claim, this was a more relaxed conversation. In saying that his "habits" might go away without his doing anything about them, he was really saying that he was ready to let them go. And as a matter of fact he was more ready to leave the therapeutic relationship. The words he used were the same as he had used many times before but the feeling he expressed was different.

In talking of doctors Solomon differentiated his present doctor from the others. Once as he was quoting the "doctor" the therapist commented: "You don't think of me as a doctor." He agreed that he did not and said: "You call the nurse a social worker and you are a psychiatrist—not a doctor." Both smiled and agreed that this was a strange and different place. His own growing feeling of difference at this point gained meaning through contrast, and this comparison provided him with an objective means of measuring his new sense of adequacy.

There were regret and some belligerence in his statement: "My mother worries mostly about my brother now." His own difference from his brother was better established but the mother's shifting emphasis, which was quite apparent in her interviews with the social worker, brought to Solomon the awareness of what he had given up and of what his "sick" brother was now receiving.

This led to a further discussion of ending. Solomon introduced the time question: "When I come to a place I want to get well in a day." "I know that, Solomon, and now you are about ready to stop." "Yes, I wouldn't come here for a year more." Again the therapist agreed and joked with him a little by saying, "I'd throw you out before that time." This boy who had been so intense and serious in everything he did was relieved by this light human quality of the therapist and smiled and said he did not want to come much longer and immediately referred with a touch of his own humor to the ten doctors he had seen who had said they could get him well. They laughed together as they talked about his attempt to add one more to his list of victims. Solomon felt relief that he had not succeeded.

At the end of this hour the therapist commented that he had observed that Solomon never showed his tics when he was with the therapist. With a surprised look he replied: "I thought I did. I only shake when I think about it." The therapist responded, "And when you don't think about it you just go ahead being Solomon and not a dish of jello." The hearty laughter which followed was the most genuine response this boy had ever given.

In the fifteenth hour Solomon was ready to discuss a plan for ending but he approached this negatively. He wanted to paint but said, "There are no paints," and, "There is no paper." To this the therapist commented: "Sounds as if you don't think there is much here you want and you probably are about finished." He agreed but he was finding it hard to take a definite step toward ending. He made two statements which revealed the dilemma so commonly found in the ending experience. One was, "I can't stop coming." He balanced this with, "Yes. I am ready to stop, I can hardly wait. I wish it were today." Then he brought out, to support the first feeling, "I still am afraid to go to bed when the lights are out." This statement had little to do with the behavior at home but had a great deal to do with the anxiety that was awakened by his readiness to end. He went ahead, however, and talked about the oldest brother and of his strong desire to live there "because then I would have no fear. I could go to bed without a light and not be bothered at all." The termination of treatment led to Solomon's reaching out increasingly for the support that he felt existed in this brother, a support which he was leaving in his relationship to the therapist. No ten-year-old boy can grow without some supporting framework from the adult world. It was this that Solomon needed as he continued to find himself in the realities of his everyday living.

That treatment hour concluded with his decision to use the next time to settle on a definite ending date. In the meantime Solomon could talk it over with his mother. She was an important factor in the decision to end treatment, and since she was ready for it also, she could give real support to her son who could not get to that same point all by himself.

The next hour was an important one. It brought out the striking difference between talking about ending and experiencing the meaning of ending. Solomon started with some anxiety, and wanted again to play checkers, saying, "I can beat several fellows bigger than myself." This expressed his acceptance of his own ability, and not his brother's.[6] As he was preparing the board he was reminded of last week's decision to get something important settled today. He stalled

---

[6] It will be recalled that when Solomon played checkers in the second hour he was identified with his "sick" brother and relied on this brother's prowess in checkers to play his own game.

and asked "what?" The therapist suggested he answer that and he made two totally irrelevant guesses. The therapist commented that Solomon was finding it hard to settle down and act on his readiness to end. He said nothing more but he played two good games of checkers.

The question of termination was reopened by the therapist who commented on Solomon's anxiety in facing this question. He tried to reassure himself and asked: "What is there to be afraid of?" The therapist replied: "Because you are not quite sure you can hold the feeling of being well that you have gained right here." He assented, saying, "I wouldn't be sure I would be well." The therapist agreed to the risk involved, and that ending would and did activate that uncertainty. With some help Solomon then settled on four more appointments. He was intrigued and relieved with this decision and talked about what he had missed at school through coming here. When the therapist suggested, "Suppose you call your mother on the telephone and tell her of your decision," his first impulse was to do this. As he made the move to pick up the telephone, however, he retreated from this daring act. With a little encouragement he went ahead, asked for his mother, and before she answered he exclaimed: "Gee—I'm scared." When his mother answered, timidly he asked: "Mother, how much longer shall I come?" The therapist broke in and said: "Solomon, you're just trying to get your mother to decide what you have really decided." So he blurted out: "I am coming four more times." She thought that was fine, and a look of the most intense relief was on Solomon's face as he hung up, saying in a surprised tone, "She said it was all right." As he wiped the perspiration from his forehead the therapist casually said, "That was kind of scarey." Without any qualification and with great relief he said, "I was scared but when I went ahead and did it, it was not so hard." The therapist added: "Solomon, in the past when you have been scared of doing something you would not go ahead, and would use being scared as an excuse for not doing it. You found just now, just as you found when you first came, that when you go ahead, even though scared, that the fear disappears." When he left a few minutes later he was a relaxed and natural ten-year-old boy and repeated: "I was scared but it wasn't so hard after all." He had again learned the difference between talking and doing, between talking about feeling and experiencing it.

The next week Solomon had a cold and was not able to come to the clinic. Ending had aroused considerable anxiety and prior to the hour just described, he had been more difficult at home. This was the temporary exaggeration of symptoms commonly observed around ending, both in children and adults, which frequently is misunderstood as evidence of the patient's needing more help.

In his next hour Solomon was quite at ease. The therapist raised the question of making up the missed hour, since they had settled on four, but left the decision about this entirely with Solomon. He could not decide, so around his trying to settle this point he and the therapist again discussed his feeling about ending. He brought out again his uncertainty of remaining well. There was no effort on his part to deny his anxiety nor was he using his feeling as a weapon to extend his time. There was a healthier meeting and handling of his anxiety as Solomon and the therapist talked about the similarity of the feeling he had when he started treatment to the feeling he had now as he was ending. He took an active part in this discussion.

In the next to the last hour Solomon announced: "I have decided next time will be the last." Not only had he taken the responsibility of this decision, but, in doing so, he gave up an hour that he could have had. The content of the whole hour was on what he was doing at school and in the neighborhood. Actually, he was doing many more things and doing them well, and in sharing his satisfaction in these achievements, he was also sharing the evidence of his assumption of self-responsibility for them. There was no struggle in this and in every way he indicated his feeling of being through with treatment.

Solomon described his last hour as "exciting," and talked more about his "face movements." For the first time he demonstrated the nature of the movements. The therapist met this by saying: "Solomon, you are saving a few things to work on and correct all by yourself after you end." He agreed as he recognized the conscious control he had over these movements. The only excess facial movement he showed was during the demonstration. He also said, "I am all over those fears, but I am a little afraid of stopping," and he talked of the possibility of returning sometime "for a visit."

Solomon spent the last hour on his favorite checkergame. He played an excellent game and won. The second game was a draw. He was not comfortable about this and wanted a third game commenting: "If we don't, you won't have a chance to win." The therapist's saying that did not matter failed to satisfy him. So a third game followed and he made little effort to win. He had to end by not winning a game and this carried great meaning around the bigger game he had struggled to win. He had won a greater victory by finding he could begin to use his energies for growth.

A small but significant thing happened in the waiting room at the end of this last hour. The mother had always fussed with Solomon's coat collar each time they left the clinic to go home. That act symbolized her relationship to this boy. On this day his zipper stuck and he worked to get his collar fastened around his neck. She stood by and let him fix it. It was a small thing but it showed the extent of her movement away from being a worrying, fussing, overanxious person to the point where she was free to be the mother of a growing boy.

Several months after ending the mother reported that Solomon was getting along quite well. A few of his facial tics remained but she expressed little concern about them and felt they were gradually disappearing.

7

PROBLEMS ARISING IN WORKING WITH AGGRESSIVE BEHAVIOR

CHILDREN WITH dominantly aggressive behavior present many challenging problems to the therapist. These children have been in conflict with all forms of authority. Their relationships with parents and teachers and other children are built around attempts to level the controls others try to exercise. While on the surface these children give the impression of great strength and arrogance and of being afraid of nothing, actually they are, as a rule, children who are quite fearful and uncertain. They are afraid of any yielding since that involves giving in and using the strength of another rather than trying to eliminate the natural authority which is a part of all living. They are afraid of the more gentle, positive type of feeling expression as this involves sharing and being related to another person on a basis of growth rather than on a basis of control.

I am presenting a second case in detail for two major reasons. First, this boy's interviews illustrate vividly many details of and problems arising in the therapeutic process. Second, a psychiatrist in training worked with this boy and the material brings out the way in which a therapist can learn through doing. The material also throws into relief some of the common difficulties a therapist encounters and indicates how these can be met without blocking the essential movement of the child.

The outward difficulties of seven-year-old Jimmy were manifest in his negatively aggressive behavior at school where "he will not work," and in his determination to have "what he wants when he wants it." Underneath these assertive demands the mother described him as a "timid, unhappy, and easily frightened child."

Jimmy's mother was a sober, somewhat prim person in her early thirties. She was completely absorbed in her efforts to be an adequate mother and wife. She had developed few interests outside of her home and was inclined to take on herself the responsibility for everything that went wrong, not only with her son but with her husband. The death of her first child at the age of four had left her burdened with the conviction that she had been responsible for his death. This reinforced her tendency to carry the burden of Jimmy's difficulties. She was closely bound to him by her effort to atone for the guilt she felt in the death of her first child and her attempts to mold into a different form, and to correct Jimmy's emerging behavior difficulties, were continuous and increasingly futile.

The discussion of this case will emphasize the boy's material. But, as I have previously indicated, it should be kept constantly in mind that the mother, with the help of a skilled social case worker, was making considerable progress in breaking up her too complete and unreal sense of responsibility. She initiated the first step in this direction when she brought her son to the clinic and thus allowed him to share some responsibility in the problem. The acceptance of the value of and necessity for his active participation in therapy was her first recognition of his part in the creation of the problem. This left the mother freer to work on the part that really belonged to her, and was a step in the direction of her becoming the boy's mother and not the all-enveloping life force that she was attempting to be for him with such discouraging results. Both mother and boy were involved in this problem and, in coming to the clinic, both participated in bringing about a different balance in their relationship to each other and to themselves. Keeping in mind the importance of the mother's part in therapeutic work with children, we can now proceed to a detailed discussion of the child's material.

In his first hour with the psychiatrist, Jimmy left his mother without hesitation. His rapid and tense talk provided but a thin veneer to the fear aroused in him by this new adventure. In his talk he told of his interest in drawing: "I could make a sketch of our house," but he did not get around to this until he had told about his club and the fights they have. He built his house with the clay and, on this more familiar ground, he became much freer. He talked about the house and how he might become an architect, putting all his uncertainty on the future as he said: "I can't decide what I want to be." He was helped back to more immediate realities by the therapist's comment that he might decide what he could do and be right now. To this he responded: "Yes, if I want to, it's whatever you can get, isn't it?" This was Jimmy's opening shot.

He worked hard in completing his "house" and at the end of the hour helped with putting things away. The therapist discussed with Jimmy the possibility of his coming each week at this same hour and told him about the length of each appointment. Jimmy was interested and accepted the suggestion of the therapist that he write his name on the calendar for his next appointment. He volunteered, as they were returning to the waiting room, "I like this place." In this first hour he had made the place his own and was off to a rapid start, as we can see more clearly in his second hour, when

Jimmy was less tense and eager to get started. He took the leadership not only in the hour itself but also in his description of how he came to the clinic. "I had to get my mother up, she knew I was coming but I had to get her up." In his manner and conversation he was trying to be more like an adult than a child and talked about "when I was a child," and, "how nice it is to have someone to talk to." He was handling the beginning of this experience by erasing his difference between himself and his doctor. This is a commonly occurring phenomenon with children who throw themselves into an experience with such completeness.

He told more about his club saying, "I'm quitting the club and getting up one of my own. Those boys aren't very nice. They're always telling me 'You're out or you're in' and I don't like people telling me what to do." Jimmy conveyed in these statements several important meanings to his therapist. He expressed his intention to continue coming to this "new club." But in doing this he temporarily disowned "the bad" in himself and portrayed the boys he was leaving in his old club as possessing that quality. In addition, he was establishing a foundation for controlling this new experience, and made it clear that he was the organizer of it and that he did not intend to have anyone telling him what to do. He was going to be the boss and thus control what might go on. The therapist made no comments about these remarks, and he went on to say with real assertion: "I'm going to make 'em do what I want. I'll get back at them and trip up their plans and will they be mad, and if you have good ideas, you let me have them." In this way Jimmy included the therapist in this new venture he was undertaking and felt free to use and demand her ideas and strength. This was an important and necessary use of the therapist at this point.

Jimmy became engaged in a phantasy play between Indians and soldiers. "The soldiers will be mean to the Indians, they will capture them and make them slaves, they'll use them plenty." The boy seemed to sense the need to preserve some secrecy about his intentions and changed his play saying, "You don't know what I'm going to make." Thus he reasserted his own separateness which the therapist could support by saying, "You're right, not unless you tell me." He then wanted to know more about the therapeutic situation and asked: "How long do I stay here altogether?" "We have forty-five minutes, Jimmy." He protested: "That doesn't count up to much." He admitted that he wanted more time, but what he really wanted was to test out who was in control. So when he said, "As long as I am here, I want either an hour or less than forty-five minutes," he was finding, out of the reality which time gave, that he had to adapt to a limit and fit into a plan determined by the necessities of this new situation.

It may seem arbitrary to those who have not worked with children to hold to a time schedule. However, a known situation provides an important opportunity for the child to struggle against the control of the real limits imposed by this new experience. While these limits are defined by the therapist, they are not a personal exercise of power. A therapist who accepts fully the responsibility implicit in his role must give definition to that role by holding the child to the limits which, in reality, are binding both upon him and upon the child. There is real meaning in helping a child to bring into the open the feeling roused in him by his encountering a limit. In this way, the fixed and static fact of time takes on dynamic meaning through the struggle the child puts into controlling it. This boy showed and admitted some anger, particularly in his vehement denial that he wanted to do anything about it, saying: "I'm not the boss, I don't own this place so it's not up to me to set the time." The therapist was prompt in making good use of this in her comment: "While you can't be the boss on time, you can be the boss in deciding what to do in the time you have." Jimmy looked astonished and with relief said: "I'm sure glad I met you." There is real relief for these aggressive children who find that they can express their anger aroused by a limitation with a person who, while being firm, can, at the same time, encourage the expression of that feeling.

This [1] hour concluded with an interesting play phantasy. Jimmy made a clay wagon and assumed the role of driver. The therapist suggested that she would like a ride. "All right, I will take a doctor and a nurse in the cart, they balance each other and are made of the same stuff." In this play, he was the driver and the controlling force but he could not allow the doctor to be a person in her own right. The comments made by the therapist were wisely related to the content of the play. It was necessary for him to end the hour with the resumption of some of the control he had given up in accepting the time limit. He wrote his name on the calendar for his next appointment but refused the proffered pencil saying, "I got a pencil of my own in my pocket."

In this second hour Jimmy, who had thrown himself into this experience with such completeness, was beginning to find, not in words nor in interpretations, but through experience, what he could be in this new relationship. His first responses indicated a rather complete identification with the therapist, which would be threatening unless he could be in control. He was beginning to test that out, and in doing so was taking his first step in finding what he could be and what the therapist could be with him. Growth, whether in its natural setting or in the unique setting of a therapeutic relation, cannot take place in a vacuum. It is a living phenomenon. It involves assertion and yielding, and just as the doctor

[1] For a full discussion of the time element in therapy, cf. Taft, Jessie, *op. cit.*, ch. I.

and the nurse balanced each other in Jimmy's play cart, so Jimmy will have to find that yielding and assertion must balance each other in his living experiences with others.

In evaluating a child's progress through his successive therapeutic hours, a realization of his basic movement is of more significance than absorption with the detailed content of each hour. In other words, the growing evidence of differentiation in the course of the child's therapeutic experience must be the therapist's primary basis of orientation. In the case under discussion, the child's movement can be more clearly followed if this is kept in mind.

In the third hour Jimmy arrived in a vigorous mood announcing, "There is a bomb in this room today, right in my pocket." The bomb was actually in his assertive feeling and probably related to his anticipated need to maintain the control which he was in danger of losing following the too complete absorption of the first two hours. But he did not act like a bomb. Instead he was uncertain in his choice of activity, balanced the merits of making things with wood or cardboard, of drawing or painting, and this vacillation culminated in his saying, "It's hard to tell what I would do—I do the funniest things." Jimmy agreed to his difficulty in making up his mind and added, "That is hard, I need some help in making up my mind."

This boy was in a dilemma common to children in the early stages of therapy. The freedom to decide on their own activity at this point is determined by the amount of responsibility they can take for being themselves. Jimmy, as is true with most children needing help, brought to the therapist this uncertain and inadequate feeling about himself which emerged from the dilemma created by the desire to be all-powerful in the face of his need for dependence. He figuratively swallowed the therapist in his first two hours. She was incorporated as an undifferentiated part of himself, and this stirred both anxiety and a feeling of safety. To decide things for himself would, in effect, be saying, "I don't need you, I am capable of living my own life." That horn of the dilemma is balanced by the other which, in effect, says, "I can't do anything without you, so you decide." There is greater safety and more control in the latter. The child who is struggling against accepting responsibility for himself may center his fight on the choice of activity and, by deciding nothing for himself, try to make the therapist carry the burden. One boy of eight carried this struggle to the extreme of asking after several interviews, "Which chair shall I sit in?" Some adults mistakenly call this politeness.

Jimmy could admit and accept some need for help. What constituted help at this point was an important and puzzling question. The beginning student commonly makes either the mistake of passive inaction, which fails to give the support necessary, or of doing too much and carrying too much responsibility. Neither reaction provides the help the child needs. Real help lies in being with the child as he fumbles along his journey of self-discovery. Such a concept rests upon a base of respect for the child's capacity eventually to work through to a more responsible use of himself. Words and action are not so important as the quality a therapist can express in this relationship by his manner, his natural and unobtrusive friendliness, and to which children are more apt to respond.

Jimmy reacted in a characteristic way, even before the therapist could say anything. He sensed that his asking for help brought him too close to her and he immediately took on the "pretend" character of the radio comedian, "Rochester." "I'm Rochester, I got to go and see my boss to see what I can do next week." When the therapist could ask, "What's the matter with seeing what he can do right now?" she allowed the phantasy character to remain but brought Jimmy back to the immediate reality of the hour. With that support, and in the partial isolation of a phantasy role, he decided to build a house, and sustained for the balance of the hour the first creative activity initiated by himself.

Through this crucial point in the case, the therapist had been oriented to the child's underlying capacity for positive action. It is easy to lose that base by being drawn into the child's more obvious and more immediate negative expressions. There was less danger of that with Jimmy than with many children, but in the case of Solomon (Chapter VI) the determined effort of the boy to maintain his irresponsible position was more persistent and glaringly apparent.

This boy captured, for the few remaining minutes of his third hour, a more responsible feeling about himself. It was transitory but yet so important that he wanted to do all he could with it while it lasted. He worked hard on his building and anxiously said: "I hope my time is not up before I get this finished." He needed the tangible evidence of a completed house to give more substance to the fleeting creative quality which had been so elusive in his life up to this point. This represented another step in Jimmy's differentiating himself from the therapist. Even though he needed the role of Rochester to get started, he carried on as Jimmy. The development and sustaining of the new quality in himself that came to life in this hour is the essence of what we call therapy. How Jimmy maintained and broadened, or attempted to deny or exaggerate, this more alive feeling about himself will now be traced through his subsequent hours.

A further comment about the nature of Jimmy's play may amplify and clarify points made in an earlier chapter on the value of play. Jimmy might well have chosen other play media with the same meaning. The really dynamic value of his play was not in what he chose but rather in his freedom at that time to initiate something within the framework of a relationship where his vacillation and uncertainty were accepted, and where he could be helped to risk a more positive expression of himself. The real value of these therapeutic hours would have been sidetracked and lost had the therapist sought to find, in the play itself, hidden historic meanings. To do that would be foreign to the concept of therapy I am presenting in this book.

In the fourth hour, the house still held great meaning for Jimmy. He was pleased to find it still there in the therapist's office, and said: "I told my mother it would be here, but she said it wouldn't with all the children who come here." Actually, this was his own doubt. Frequently it is not possible to save what a child begins to make as it would involve putting false restrictions on the activity of other children using the room. To try too hard to save such material represents a too-protective attitude toward the child, in the therapist's assumption that the child is not capable of handling the disappointment and anger that would be stirred up. If this house had been destroyed by another child, it would have been necessary for the therapist to use that reality to help the child express his resentment and to begin again, possibly in a medium that had more permanence than blocks on the floor of an office used by many other children.

Jimmy said with intensity. "This is going to be a hard job," and he was right because the house really carried so much of his own creative impulse. The student therapist made the common mistake of remarking on the negative implications in such a statement as this, and suggested that he did not want to do anything hard. This interpretation was only a half-truth, even though Jimmy continued in his efforts to shift the responsibility of his self-initiated activity and kept asking for suggestions as to what he should do next. He was neither ready nor willing to detach this new quality in himself from the therapeutic relationship in which he was discovering it. As he went intently ahead he kept talking, partly to himself, but also to the therapist: "You got to concentrate on this, you gotta figure out how it goes for yourself, you gotta be smart to do this." When he reached a difficult place in the construction he said: "I think I could stand a little help on this." Help was given and the boy went on with more confidence, and in a more demanding tone said, "You better get some good mortar for this."

At this point Jimmy did an interesting thing. Suddenly he destroyed the whole house and with real relief laughed and talked about knocking it down. Then he started to build again with greater ease and confidence. The meaning of this destructive act seemed clear. He had built that house within the supporting framework of this relationship. The therapist had to supply the "mortar" that held it up. As it grew it was a house created not by himself but by the communal self that he tried to maintain in his relationship to the therapist. The destruction was a necessary step in starting over in order to get more sense of his own creative effort in building the house, a symbol of himself. He used the help of the therapist but, in doing so, became doubtful of his own effort and the value he could place on it. The building of the house, the destruction and the new start all were concrete manifestations of this boy's problem. In four interviews he had brought his whole growth problem into this new experience and was able to express in these hours the struggles and anxieties that made up so much of his life with his mother. While he destroyed the house, he retained the start he had made toward a new and creative use of his own capacity.

Jimmy rebuilt the house with renewed zeal and soon it became more than a house. It became a place to live in and he talked about who would live in it. The house had taken on that living quality as he gained more sense of himself in what he was doing. His activity was more spontaneous and he sang while he built and said, "I'm a funny person." But he was a person, that was the important new development for him. He began to put more detail into the new structure and could not decide where the different rooms belonged or whether to have a door. He decided not to have a door but to let the house be "free for all." He was not ready to own the house and have it belong to specific people, nor could he allow himself at this point to live in it with a particular person. He was not ready to differentiate himself to that extent.

At this point he asked for more help. "I want someone to decide things, will you decide?" The therapist was properly concerned with his fumbling efforts to make decisions and commented on the feeling that was evident, but she did not jump in with help. Jimmy became more demanding but finally reached the point when he could say, "Maybe I can decide." In his uncertainty he fumbled through to a decision but he had to make further efforts to shift the responsibility to the therapist who was concerned primarily with the feeling that was aroused and not with the particular thing he was building.

A week later Jimmy began right where he had stopped the preceding week and asked for his house which in the interim had been taken down by another child. This fact opened a new opportunity for helping. That house was the objectification of a self Jimmy could not fully own. Its removal made it necessary for him to rely more on what he had gained in himself through building the house. His first reaction was to cover up the feeling aroused by this loss. The therapist commented on his probable anger but reassuringly he said, "It's all right, I figured on doing something else." However, he just wandered about the office and was unnaturally sweet saying, "I'm glad I came, I'm glad I got to know you." There was some discussion of why he came and he put all the burden on "my trouble doing arithmetic." But he expressed some anger and complained about "not having enough time to play." Again he began to demand that he be told what to do and in this way was able to express more openly his anger over having his house taken down. When the therapist again commented on this he said, "Maybe I don't feel like telling you." This was a real assertion for Jimmy and carried the force of a feeling he no longer had to deny by covering it up with sweetness.

The change in Jimmy was immediate. He asked for paper, remarking, "I think I might paint," and he was helped to get started. His restlessness disappeared along with his strained, unhappy facial expression. He painted a red fire engine and told of a radio program about ghosts. "It really made me afraid at night then." The therapist related this to the more immediate concern he had in making up his own mind and to this he gave an emphatic, "Yes ma'am." In the remainder of the hour he could ask for help without demanding it and at the end said, "We are getting somewhere now." With more relaxation he added: "I'm not really going to finish this. I'm in no hurry to get it home."

When a child is just making the start described in these five hours, it may seem strange to talk about the first evidence of ending. But it ceases to be strange if ending is understood as a phase in the process of achieving a separate self. By reviewing the nature of this problem at the beginning and the movement up to this point, we can see implications for ending in Jimmy's last remark. At the start this boy and his mother were deadlocked in a negative struggle. His mother was determined to be the "good mother" who smoothed the way for a boy who persistently demanded but made little creative use of all the mother was impelled to give. She carried so much of his responsibility for living, and as long as he could maintain that life force in her he could avoid creative use of his own efforts to achieve a self of his own.

In this dilemma they sought help and the boy swallowed, figuratively speaking, the therapist, room, and all. Thus he sought to make the therapist carry the load he had previously placed on his mother. But, in four therapeutic hours, he began to find a new use of himself. At first there was anxious urgency to utilize fully this impulse while he had it. As he became a little more certain of holding this creative feeling he settled into a more relaxed tempo and was in no hurry to take himself out of this growth-inducing experience. There was an awareness of a new sense of a self, separate and apart from the therapist. Each move that he now made toward a clearer definition and use of his own ability was a step toward ending eventually his experience with the therapist.[2]

About this time the mother presented important background material as a part of her own movement in becoming more real in her role as mother. The mother again referred to her first child who had died at the age of four, told how she had protected that child from every possible danger and how she had been unable to risk letting her have any life of her own, fearing the child might have to face the hardships she had met in her own development. In the child's death she described both sorrow and relief, but she felt keenly a punishment for not having allowed the child to have more part in her own living. The patient was her second child. She was determined to make him more responsible and found herself locked in the struggle that prevented attainment of the very goal she sought.[3] She was making progress at this point,

[2] The dynamics of the ending phase are discussed fully in Chapter IX.
[3] This is a common dilemma that grows out of a parent's desire and effort to *give* responsibility to a child. No one can do that for another human being. Responsibility is an emergent feeling that defines a person's attitude and use of himself. A parent can guide and define the conditions in which a child can become responsible, but he can never *make* a child feel responsible.

Adolf Meyer, *op. cit.*, p. 26, had this in mind when he said: "By the person's spontaneity I mean that which the person may be expected to

in living, for the first time, her role as a mother and she described considerable improvement in the boy. She was beginning to accept the fact that Jimmy had a part in the creation of his problem. She no longer had to carry the whole responsibility for his difficulties, and she could let him have a real part in working out their solution. By giving up a part of the problem to the boy she could begin to acquire a more responsible acceptance of her own part in it. Sometimes cases in a child guidance clinic break off at this point when a parent, facing that realization, is not able to take that next step but ends his clinic contact by resuming the old way of living.

When Jimmy arrived for his sixth hour, he was excited. Entering the same room as before, he said: "This is the highest I've ever been up. It's pretty far up here." His growth felt both exciting and frightening to him. He sat in his little chair and announced: "I need ten cents and five kids. I want to wire for a telephone and then members of my club could talk to each other." Thus he diluted the exciting nature of this experience with the phantasy of its being a club. He was ready for a more direct medium of communication. The therapist suggested that if he had such a system, he could more easily talk about the things that bothered him. This emphasized a particular content that represented the therapist's interest. Jimmy evaded the issue raised, and continued in his own way.

He returned to his painting of the fire engine and finished it with the addition of several fire extinguishers "on this truck of ours." He was playing safe. He took some new paper, announced, "I am going to surprise you," and drew the outlines of a boat, then demanded, "You are going to tell me what this is." He was more anxious than controlling, and

---

rise to and to rise with on his own, 'sua sponte' with his 'spons' and 'response' and finally 'responsibility.' "

the therapist simply and wisely responded: "It's a boat." He agreed with pleasure and relief.

Jimmy was puzzled as for the first time now he raised the question as to why he "comes and just plays." The therapist could have responded to this by saying that he came now because he wanted to and thus affirm his responsibility, not only for coming, but for his activity during the hour. Instead she responded in terms of a problem, saying that some children did nothing but play, while others talked and did something about things that worried them. This was too vague and too remote to have much meaning for Jimmy. But when the therapist referred to his difficulty in making up his own mind, she struck a more immediate reality and he answered with a vigorous demand that he be told what to do.

Children are quick to respond to the real and present sources of difficulty and equally quick to find a safe medium to work them out. Jimmy looked into all of the drawers saying, "I don't know what drawers to look in first. There are so many in this darn place. Now tell me. Come on. Ladies first. You do what I say for once." But he continued what he had started and looked in every drawer and closet. The therapist was not clear about the meaning of this activity but it became clearer when Jimmy found a hammer and said, "This is my idea. I might make something if it didn't make too much noise." He wanted to go ahead with his own idea, but it was a little dangerous and he sought support for his activity. He postponed action saying, "I could bring wood the next time and make something." The therapist met this evasion and said, "How about doing something now?" and with that help he made a small beginning toward carrying out his idea as the hour ended.

Through the type of struggle found in this hour, the boy moved toward a definition of a self he could experience in relationship to another. Enmeshed as he had been in a negative expression of himself, there would naturally be this testing out before he could be free to live positively. This involved sharing which, to a negative and hostile child, means loss of self. Hostile feelings serve as a protective barrier against the loss the individual fears from a more positive relationship.

An air of mystery was introduced by Jimmy in his seventh hour. He carried on the mysterious search through the drawers that he had begun in his previous hour. A nest of dolls was found and it held "a secret no one is to know." He seemed more sure of himself and there was different purpose in his moves. He proceeded to take over the office as his own but complained: "You have so many things but you don't have what I want." He was certainly trying to find a place for this newly acquired self which did not entirely fit into this new relation. He was as puzzled about his growing sense of difference.

Having fixed "his office" he proceeded to telephone his therapist but could not think of a name to give her in the new role he assigned to her. He had always called her Doctor but now changed this to Mrs. and asked, "Will you come over to my office and see me?" He had taken over the role of doctor and gave many reasons why he could not come to the therapist's office saying, finally, "The only way for me to see people is for them to come and see me." "Could we talk on the phone?" was the therapist's suggestion. "No, I have to *see* you, to show you some things, and I am going on a fishing trip." So the therapist played out the role and pantomimed her arrival. Jimmy then phoned the boss and said, "Dr. X is coming to see me, anything you want to talk over with her?" He had the boss reply, "No, you can handle all the business." Jimmy was trying to be the boss and at the same time to divest himself of the role.

Jimmy carried through the phantasy and announced: "I have something important to do in this world." Then he asked for advice about the best fishing places and said: "You know more about that than I do," but "some day I am going to know how to catch all sorts of fish." The therapist expressed an interest in what the present seven-year-old Jimmy could catch. He overlooked this and again phoned, asking for "the boss" and in response the therapist suggested that he was the boss and that she was there to see him. This aroused some guilt and brought him back to a more realistic basis. "I'm afraid I can't be the boss." He said he could not be the boss of those "lousy kids at home," but "I'm going to boss it into them, I am boss, I need some practice." He engaged in some active building, and asked timidly, "Do you like noise?" He was encouraged to make a little and find out. "In some ways I like to make noise and in some ways I don't." In this way he expressed the uncertainty aroused by his change. He was in need of the "practice" provided by each hour with his therapist where he could experience these conflicting feelings of assertiveness and yielding.

In the fourth chapter the important problem of the therapist's active participation in the child's play was discussed. This problem became a real one here as the child was requiring of the therapist active dramatization of herself in a new role. A therapist must keep constantly in mind the need of remaining the therapist. He would cease to be this if he were pushed into one role or another by the shifting demands of the child. The essential foundation for the differentiating process would be destroyed without a steady quality that preserved in the therapist his own integrity. Therefore in this instance there was no help to the boy in the therapist's playing out the role of one being bossed. It only made Jimmy guilty and led to his saying, "I'm afraid I can't be the boss." It would have been better if the therapist had maintained her therapeutic role and had helped the boy to continue his play through her interest rather than through active participation.

Jimmy seemed aware of reaching a critical place in this experience when he came in his next hour and solemnly announced: "There are lots of puzzling things on my mind. I've got to stay a long time to get them all straight." The therapist suggested they get right at them and he said, "It's about those button things downstairs with wires—how do they work?" The therapist missed the point of this entirely when she said there were more important things than that to work on. In response, Jimmy became evasive and, in fussing with some wood, said, "You will have to guess what this is going to be." But he made it clear that it was a sign he was making saying, "You will know what this one means if you know what signs mean." Then he put "R.R." on it. The therapist misinterpreted the meaning of this because of her preoccupation with the negative impulse in this boy and said, "It looks like a danger sign—don't go ahead. You might get too close to your troubles." Jimmy was astonished and quickly said, "No." He agreed that it was a railroad sign but added, "Last week I didn't know it would be one. It would not be a railroad sign if it meant keep out of any troubles."

The boy was right. The therapist got on the wrong track at the beginning of the hour with her preoccupation with his symptoms at home. His concern with telephone wires in his opening remark referred to his immediate relationship with the therapist. He had a beginning awareness of his own separateness but needed a medium of communication, not to convey any particular problem but to maintain a connection with the source of so much that was new and strange in himself. The telephone provided a safe means of communication between himself and the therapist. He could convey his meaning to her without being either too close or too remote.

In this case, the boy was not thrown off the track, and it was quite possible that the therapist's failure to sense his meaning required him to make a clearer statement. He was talking, of course, about ending, and the railroad interest symbolized the separation feeling which he proceeded to clarify further. He was full of his plans for the future, a thing he had never dared to do before. He would make four or five signs he said, and "Then I'll bring a new bag and each week I'll have a new sign to take home." The interest he now showed in the other boys who came to see the therapist was not one that excluded them, but more the interest of including himself in what they did. He was in possession of a beginning new self-realization but he still needed the pattern that all growing children need. So when he asked what the other boys did there was more desire to use their activities to fashion his own, rather than to imitate their actions to avoid the responsibility for his own growing feeling of difference. The therapist, however, correctly maintained her interest in Jimmy as a part of the support that she could give to him as he moved toward a fuller achievement of his own separate self.

Jimmy was finding the movement in this direction both exciting and frightening. As he made one of his signs and nailed it up in plain view, he said, "I'm glad to do that because I have never done it before. I don't want to do it and yet I do." He saw an ediphone cylinder, asked about its use and when told, said, "If I had it, I'd put my whole life on it. But I can't give my whole life to another person I don't trust." He was sober here and the therapist talked with him about the difficulties in trusting anyone with so much. He added, "I can trust you but you live too far away. If you lived closer, I could run wires to you. I don't want to be too close to you."

It was not the therapist he distrusted, but rather this new awareness of his separateness, his new ownership of a self that was not bound up in another person. This feeling of his individuation was exciting, but the movement away from the therapist was frightening, re-creating the old desire to get back to an earlier safety that stemmed from dependence. So his statement, "But I don't want to be too close," summed up his need for a communicating connection in order to maintain the partial support he still needed. At the end of the hour when he let the therapist have the secret number it was as if he had said: "I can trust my new self to you." He could do that without the old fear of losing his whole self. Jimmy left that hour with confidence, saying, "It's fun to play here."

In this next hour, the ninth, he was eager and full of plans. First Jimmy wanted to make more signs, but then changed to painting and became enthusiastic about finger painting. "It is so gushy, you can't tell which way it is going." He became quite mysterious as he said: "Three people know me —myself, the doctor and a third. We don't know where he is, but he is here. He has power no one else has." Then he asked the therapist to name this unknown force. It seemed quite clear that this unknown represented the new Jimmy whom he could not as yet own fully but had to maintain as a mysteriously powerful force. It was not particularly helpful when the therapist guessed that it was God. However, Jimmy was delighted to have an identity for this magic that allowed him to keep it outside of himself. He went on talking about magic and when in mixing two colors he made brown, he was ecstatic. "See, I've discovered something. I can make a magic carpet. It's like magic, you could be an artist and know everything that is going on." He went on talking about mysterious messages and about wires not being connected. The therapist suggested that he might send a message that could be understood, but he continued to be evasive, saying, "I must practice my abc's." He agreed with the therapist that he had found a good place to get that practice.

While giving an external identity to the newness in himself, Jimmy was experimenting to find out how much of the "magic" he could accept as his own. For many children, and also for adults, it seems like magic when they find an easier, a less struggling and a more positive way of living. They come to a therapist fearfully and find relaxation in building a relationship with another person without placing themselves in the power of that person. It probably was this way with Jimmy. For years he had been fighting off any relationship that was established on a give-and-take basis. By refusing to make any decisions, he had been able to make his mother live for him. After a few weeks he found himself in possession of a different feeling about himself which did not have to be maintained by fight.

There was a break in the continuity of the case since Jimmy had measles, and for five weeks appointments were canceled. The fact that sickness brought an interruption at the point where the child was bringing in so much ending material was, no doubt, a coincidence with no cause-and-effect relation in this case. However, Jimmy's use of his illness put a new emphasis on ending in the first therapeutic hour he had following his recovery. In this material, the student therapist got her first real insight into the dynamic significance of the ending process. At the same time, the deep significance of the whole experience in the boy's development was re-emphasized.

Jimmy started out where he had stopped five weeks earlier, a significant point in itself. There was some reversion to the old pattern of, "You tell me what to do." He thought the room had changed and the therapist ascribed this impression to his own change. He quickly talked of many changes in himself, referred to many troubles, "too many to talk about," and told a long story about a barn burning down. Then he added: "I feel that death is coming on—that is one of my troubles." He told of giving a knife to a boy he could not trust. It is important to recall that in the hour before his illness when he was yielding to the new impulse that it was hard for him to trust, he showed his "secret" to the therapist. To give up so much of the old must have seemed like death to this boy, a feeling that probably was reinforced by the coincidental sickness. Jimmy went on to say: "I have to get that knife back and throw the blade in the fire, then there would be no death." The therapist clarified this somewhat for the boy when she said, "Jimmy, this has a lot to do with the fact you were away from here for a long time." He evaded meeting this real source of his anxiety, and in the course of his painting activity, insisted, "I want you to learn how I do this, watch carefully. I can't tell you directly. It's no longer a secret if I tell you." The therapist, participating in this, commented on the feeling of loss he seemed to have whenever he shared a secret. Jimmy gave this remarkable reply: "If you think of what I told you today about death, you will know the secret—you can find it out indirectly because I cannot tell you directly." He then encouraged her to guess the secret number. "If you are right, I will say 10S, if wrong, I will say 11K."

The therapist responded by commenting on his anxiety about sharing this inner secret which involved expressing to her the way he felt about himself. He responded with 11K, and went on talking about death, saying: "I want to die but I want to do it to someone else instead." In this statement he was expressing a beginning affirmation of his desire to live. The therapist missed this point completely in asking, "Why do you want to die?" Jimmy knew that she had misunderstood him and closed the subject by saying: "Now don't carry it too far, that's enough for today. Next time I'll bring in the news; there is no place for death today. There is always a time and place for death but this isn't it. Do you mind if I say it this way?" Children can be accurate in the most amazing way. Jimmy's whole emphasis was on living.

Jimmy continued with more discussion of the secret which he now called the "death secret." "There is more to the secret than you told me or I told you. I would be put in jail if I told you. I know no one would really put me in jail but it would be way down deep in me and I would feel I was in prison. Do you understand that?" Actually the therapist did not understand the deep significance of this material but knew that it held real meaning to him and commented on the value and importance of his keeping his secret until he felt safer in sharing it. He said at this point: "I have one idea and if it doesn't work, I'll be put in jail."

A therapist could catch the significance of this remarkable hour only by maintaining an orientation to Jimmy's development in his constantly shifting relationship to the therapeutic situation. Starting out with no confidence, he soon threw himself completely into this new experience. There he found a gradual recognition of his difference from the therapist and this new self-realization seemed like magic to him. He gained support for this new organization of himself not only from the therapist, but also from the mother who, at the same time, was becoming more able to function naturally as his mother. This movement was all a part of the ending process which aroused Jimmy's old anxiety of losing too much of his old self. This anxiety was revived in the form of his death preoccupations and guilt over the affirmation of himself as separate and different from the therapist. This was his secret which he could not affirm by himself. He needed someone with whom to share that responsibility and it was that which he meant when he said, "I can't tell you directly."

The prison symbolism was important. It represented his feeling of being caught and trapped, but it also meant safety. Jimmy and his mother had been caught in a reality that held them like a vise. In therapy the new in each of them had come to life. But in this new experience there were two conflicting factors: there was the danger of being trapped; and the desire to be trapped because of the safety it provided him. In the ending process these two factors were balanced as he was finding out what he was ready to do on his own. Jimmy reached the point where he could say: "I have one idea and if it doesn't work, I'll be put in jail." Now he was absorbed with one idea: how to live and to end the experience in which he had found a way to live. Naturally, it was risky and, if it failed, he would have to fall back on the source of safety which the therapeutic relationship represented to him. He was holding to this anchorage while he was testing out his capacity to let it go.

The evidence of guilt shown by this boy in his desire and readiness to affirm his "secret" self has already been mentioned. This became clearer through understanding his use of the therapist. In therapeutic work the therapist can allow the child to use him, through projection, to carry the incomplete and nonacceptable aspects of the self.[4] This boy used the therapist to gain a self of his own, capable of being nourished and enriched through sharing. This was in contrast to the locked up, negative relationship with people with which he started. Now he was getting ready to end this new relationship and affirm his own difference from the source of so much that had been valuable to him. His growing sense of difference was the source of his strength, but in the ending process it was, also, the source of guilt. He had used another to gain life whom now he was wanting to leave behind. It seemed wrong even to desire to be different from

[4] This is discussed in greater detail in Chapter III.

one who had given him so much help. Children feel it wrong to be different from their parents, but that becomes only a partial feeling through the continued support and encouragement of their parents who find satisfaction in guiding children to be themselves. Jimmy, too, felt too guilty temporarily to accept and to affirm his difference from the therapist, but her acceptance of his need and his right to be different was the support that helped him to go beyond his guilt.

Following this dramatic hour to which so much attention has been given, Jimmy had six meaningful hours spread over seven weeks. He returned to his next hour ready to repair all the broken toys "so anyone else who comes can use them." This might be termed "continuing to come by proxy." It also meant that he was through with them. He was full of his own strength which he had had so little practice in using creatively. He wanted to be as strong as a giant and if he were, "I could make everyone in my gang as strong as I am." He did not want his newly developing strength to isolate him from his gang. To avoid that he could give them strength and make them like him. Children find such effective ways of using their difference while maintaining their all-important sense of belonging.

Jimmy was in a more assertive mood in contrast to the restricted guilt-bound mood of the previous hour. Today it was the therapist who would be put in jail, and "I have ways of doing things, ways that are not nice to you. No one lets me do things the way I want, but I manage to do things my way." There was uncertainty back of these exaggerated statements. He was trying too hard at this point to prove that he could be free to act on his own will and be free from the determined long-standing struggle to make others provide the stimulus for his action. He was asserting his difference from the therapist but still needed the therapist's support where he was testing out his new found sense of freedom. He imitated a dog growling and remarked: "I'm getting mad, because this building is not on fire, maybe you would go to sleep, maybe you aren't alive. Maybe I wish you were not alive." But this carried him too far and he added, "Maybe I wish I weren't alive. I don't think I'm worth living."

The therapist was not sufficiently aware of the ending implications in this material. Jimmy was struggling to free himself from the source of so much that had been creative for him, and needed encouragement in his efforts to do so. In the ending phase of therapy, children frequently want to destroy, in one way or another, the source of help. Jimmy had the therapist placed in jail and had her sent away on a long journey. The inexperienced therapist sometimes becomes involved in the negative aspects of these desires and overlooks the more positive ending impulses which, as in Jimmy's case, the child has difficulty in affirming openly. The therapist in this instance was baffled by this material and found herself too concerned with the child's more aggressive, hostile feelings which thinly covered the more positive readiness to end. Ending could have taken a smoother course if the therapist had given more support to and had clarified this direction for the child.

Jimmy continued his course, however, and justified some of his anger because the therapist was taking notes. This eased the burden for him as it gave him a more objective reason for his anger. "If I get sent to war, I would raise my fist and you would be smashed. If I really wanted to get mad you would be scared. You would be sorry you had a job here." Then he added: "Some day you might not see me here but I'll be here, invisible." This statement gave an open opportunity for a simple and direct acceptance of Jimmy's readiness to end and for help with the anxiety which naturally was aroused as he moved to this final separation step. It was a serious error when, instead of giving a warm and direct response to this, the therapist brought in the fact of a holiday break for his next appointment. That precipitated much more anxiety. In the hour, Jimmy had aggressively asserted an independence he did not entirely feel, and the change in the next appointment precipitated a realization that he had gone too far in that hour. In an anxious tone he asked: "Where will you be? Would you leave me your address as I might want to write you a letter?" Instead of helping the child with the feeling that was involved in this reaction, there was a literal response to his request and another opportunity was passed by to help Jimmy deal with the anxiety of separation while yet enabling him to retain all of his readiness to end.

It is through such material that the student therapist learns to maintain an orientation to the broader threads of movement as a child progresses toward the affirmation of what he has achieved in his therapeutic experience. The therapist, in this hour more than in any other, lost that orientation and became involved in the more negative details that cloaked the underlying meaning of Jimmy's feeling. Even with her mistakes, however, the relationship with the child was on a sound basis, and there was no serious interference with the movement toward the final goal. Jimmy had two good weeks at home and, upon returning to the clinic, the mother was full of her own readiness for a happier and more real relationship with the boy.

Jimmy was in high spirits after the week's interruption. He brought a present to the therapist and then took a book from his pocket saying: "Here it is, look it over and then you will know all the secrets." There was less mystery and a more open sharing in this act. The therapist suggested that it was still hard to talk about the secrets and he reassured her saying: "You must be patient. I want to tell you but I gotta get everything fixed first." The therapist was again too literal since she was still caught in a desire to get the content of a particular secret. The readiness to show what he called the "secret" carried the real therapeutic meaning. But the therapist was closer to what he had in mind when, for the first time, she commented that he was nearly through coming here, and that that was probably his secret. His first reaction was to deny this saying, "No, it's not that," but after a moment's reflection added, "Well, it might be. I can still be sending you letters after I don't come here any more." The therapist agreed and added that after a time he might not even want to do that. He was not sure and the therapist commented about his readiness to end and that it was hard for him to believe it. This was a little too much for him and he responded by saying, "Don't bother me and I'll get things done." He wanted some support from the therapist in ending but he also wanted to do it by himself.

Jimmy ended this hour with a more animated discussion of his club and of outside activities. Throughout these therapeutic hours Jimmy had been so deeply absorbed in the feeling of each hour that he made little mention of outside activities. The changes in the content of his conversation now reflected Jimmy's broader horizon and was concrete evidence of his moving away from the therapist into his own life. He was full of interest in his father and told about his job and a trip they had taken together. This growing identification with his father was important from two points of view: first, it was the evidence of a growing relationship with the father; second, this new relationship to his father established his separation from the therapist. He was a boy now and more ready to live that role.

Jimmy made good use of play material to carry significant feelings about himself through this ending period. For example, he made signs with a lurid mixture of colors. One sign was fixed so that it would stand upright and he said: "If I want to change this sign sometime, all I have to do is to come back here and say 'I want to change my sign,' that's what I'm going to say." The sign, as in other hours, stood for the new in himself which he gradually was accepting. Accompanying this, however, there was a desire to cling to the anchorage the therapist had provided while he was finding this new quality in himself and which he might need again if his "plans" failed. He was ready to end but along with that feeling there was, as I have already emphasized, the natural anxiety associated with the separation of himself from the source of so much help. At the end of the hour, he proudly took his sign with him, making a special point of leaving by himself and agreeing that on his next trip, he would like to come up to the office by himself.

The mother was also ready to finish the clinic experience at this same period. In a clinical procedure that brings both parent and child into active participation, the interrelation between the activity of child and parent is of prime importance.[5] In this case the mother was full of her own change of attitude in relation to her boy who was settling into a more normal way of living. His school work had improved and he was more responsive to the natural demands that the mother could, with greater naturalness, make of him. It was equally if not more important that he was better able to handle the greater freedom she was allowing him.

It was through this period that the mother became worried because some of Jimmy's behavior difficulties returned. He was more irritable and demanding and she was at a loss to know what had happened to upset him again. She was helped

---

[5] Cf. Dawley, Almena, "Inter-related Movement of Parent and Child in Therapy with Children," *American Journal of Orthopsychiatry*, v. IX, no. 4 (October, 1939).

to understand that it was a common occurrence for both child and parent to be anxious around ending and that Jimmy's behavior disturbance stemmed from his anxiety. Not only was the boy worried about his need to assume responsibility for the continuation of his more mature behavior which ending requires, but the mother also had some of the same anxiety. Helping her to understand this temporary flurry, which lasted two weeks, enabled her to hold to a steadier course and to give to the boy the help he needed in this transition period. Having these facts in mind, we can understand better the meaning of his activity in these final hours.

This hour preceded the two weeks' period of difficult behavior just mentioned. Jimmy announced his intention of making a new sign and did this. The therapist introduced more directly at this point the subject of ending, and he said rather abruptly: "I am only coming two more times, there is too much other stuff to do outside to come here every week." The abruptness of this surprised the therapist. She had thought of a longer period and she told him it was not a good idea to stop too suddenly. In this way, the therapist immediately introduced her own struggle into ending. The boy, who had had such ambivalent feelings about ending, was ready to act on his own desire to leave. He acted in an impulsive way and the therapist failed to help him express the anxiety back of his impulsive decision. She could have helped him by commenting on his need to move fast but by accepting also that he was nearly ready to leave. By her suggestion of another plan, Jimmy was free to fight her plan and to avoid meeting the turmoil in himself aroused by his growing readiness to end. It was probable that some of the difficult behavior that cropped up at home was accentuated by the therapist's excessive interference.

As we have seen in the last four or five interviews, Jimmy

had been moving slowly toward ending. So his plan of ending after two more times was not so abrupt as it sounded. If he could have had from the therapist a little more definition of his movement toward an ending, the clash begun in this hour could have been avoided.

Jimmy's reaction to a slower ending was as abrupt as his decision. He merely said, "Maybe," changed the subject and concentrated on his sign. "It's got to be perfect," he insisted, and this statement again was evidence of his need to be free of all anxiety before he could end. Some of the feeling stirred by the therapist's opposition to his plan was now expressed. In the midst of his work, he looked up and said: "I'm mad, I'm mad all the time." He did not look particularly angry. The source of anger was projected on a boy friend who told lies but he added, "Don't let me ever catch you telling lies," and in his usual enigmatic way continued: "Don't tell anyone I was born in 1896." In other words, do not say I am older than I am. This reaction was discussed in terms of the approaching end of his therapy, and of the anger precipitated by the blocking of his plan. He responded by saying, "I'm coming thirty more times. I don't know the number but it all depends upon me." This brought out clearly the will struggle that was precipitated in ending. Jimmy wanted to control all the conditions, whether it was two or thirty times. He was fighting the control of another, a fact that was really complicated by the active control the therapist introduced. Jimmy's statement was too much for the therapist to understand, who said she could not follow him but said she knew there was difficulty in his taking responsibility for ending. He made one of his penetrating observations: "If you start using your mind you'll know what I'm saying. I talk in all sorts of languages." How right he was! He proceeded to talk in terms of building a house, starting with the cellar, and he stressed the amount of lumber he would need to build the steps.

Before the hour was over Jimmy again mentioned two more appointments but with less finality. "I'm going to try and stop in two weeks. Business doesn't wait and I don't wait, summer is coming." This decision should have been accepted in the way he gave it and left for a more final settlement in his next hour. Instead, the desirability of a longer time was reintroduced and the suggestion made that possibly four more visits would be better. He replied: "If I can slow it down fast enough," and as he left he added, "I'm going to try and slow her down in a fast way."

The next hour brought this ending struggle to a climax. He was preoccupied with the nest of dolls, which he kept changing around but without any comment. The therapist asked if he still felt he must end in a hurry. He evaded this question and said: "I don't want to come, my mama can come and come, but I don't want to come any more, this is the last time." This was not challenged and Jimmy became quite silly as he wandered about saying, "Me want to sleep, me want to snore, me don't want to come, me is going to snore to death." He avoided the pronoun "I" here. The therapist was serious in her discussion of how ending seemed a little like death to him, but the other side of it was that he was so ready to live and to do other things. He persisted, however: "That's the way for me to stop, that's the way me can stop snoring."

The therapist commented on Jimmy's dilemma and expressed her interest in helping him as she had helped him on other things. But he became more evasive, and with further avoidance of the "I" went on in the silly manner that thinly disguised his anxiety. "Me going to eat it up—get rid of it now." The therapist in stressing the help she was ready to give only accentuated the struggle. But he became serious as he said: "I ain't going to stop any more. I want to stop in a hurry and that is what I am going to do—you're trying to make me stay." This was true, and in his statement he clearly indicated the source of his immediate difficulty. He also defined the dilemma to the making of which the therapist had contributed. He had the compulsion to act in a hurry since he sensed the strength of his desire to keep on coming. If he did not act fast, he might not act at all. Some holding by the therapist was necessary as a means of helping him to a more solid belief in his capacity to assume the responsibilities for which he was ready. This could have been done with less control of the actual ending time had the therapist not been caught in one detail of ending, the issue of two or four times.

In this hour Jimmy talked about calling the police and putting the therapist in jail. "I'm going to get out of here today and this room will blow up in five seconds." If something could happen that would remove the therapist or the scene of their hours together, then Jimmy would be freed of the problem of how to end. The therapist's comment that that would settle his difficulty made him a little anxious, and he replied: "But I wouldn't do anything about it." He asked if there was a basement in the clinic. "I'm going to use it. I will hide there. I will board it up so no one can get in." Then he added more seriously: "I don't want to come any more. I'll burn the building down if I have to come again." Again the other side came through as he asked: "What would happen if I burned it down?" The therapist was quite helpful through this painful struggle, not so much in what was said but in her unexpressed understanding which gave the boy a feeling of support for his vacillation and for his search for a way out. She had, by this time, taken her own struggle out of it.

Jimmy made a snake out of clay and had it attack the therapist, but even as he was doing this he said: "It's up to me to decide." Even in his efforts to avoid the responsibility of his own desire, he was coming closer to accepting his own part, not only in ending, but in all that had been achieved in coming. Jimmy and the therapist were more in agreement as they looked through the calendar to settle a definite time. He said: "You write it down and I'll come if you want me to, will you be here this spring?" Yes, he was told, and this summer, too. "Can I come and see you sometime?" He was quite reassured when he was told she would be glad to have a visit from him some day.

Having yielded to his own readiness to end on a basis which he did not entirely control, Jimmy reverted to his aggressive use of the snake and made handcuffs out of clay. It was not clear whether the handcuffs were meant to hold him to the therapist or to imprison her while he got away. Both elements probably were in this behavior. But his softer feeling returned, and he wrote his name on three separate days which gave him two more appointments. He wanted to tell his mother about his decision and on the way out stopped in the office where she was talking with the social worker. The struggle was settled.

The last two hours were much easier. Jimmy announced: "It's near the end of my time here. I want to do something that counts, something to show." He prepared to paint and on returning with water said: "I just got so mad at the top of the step. I almost threw this whole can of water." But this was more of a gesture than an expression of feeling. He went ahead with elaborate preparations as "This is going to be something different. I'm experimenting. I'm just trying this out. When I end, I want to have something to show what I've accomplished." He and the therapist talked about his achievements. He enumerated a number of them and remarked: "I have learned to do many more things than before I came.

Dr. D. [he has rarely referred to her so directly by name], I've learned there are things inside of me that not even you or I know." This boy was capable of such deep understanding and had reached a point where he could allow some things to remain unknown. The human being who has to know everything and have everything explained in rational terms has never learned the peace this boy had achieved. He could accept the change in himself without having to explain it or fight against it. He could even accept the fact that his doctor did not know everything.

Jimmy was quite free in his painting and rather sloppy with the paint. This was in contrast to a rather meticulous quality that went with his earlier cautious and protective behavior. When he spilled some water he spoke of getting rid of it and added: "And I'm getting rid of this place, too." He finished two "experimental pictures." They were full of color and quite different from any he had made before. One was done rather boldly and Jimmy used his hands to spread the paint. The other was done with the brush and with fine lines. He saved both pictures to take them home and was pleased with his morning's work. In this hour, the paintings carried the satisfaction of an inner accomplishment. They told more than words could how this boy felt about being Jimmy.

In his next hour Jimmy came up to the office himself and announced: "I am not going to talk about that business." The therapist accepted this by saying that he knew what he was ready for. He agreed that was true. Again he was attracted to the bright colors in his painting and was not sure they were bright enough. He could not quite leave the ending subject alone, however, and asked: "Is this the last time I signed up for?" He was reminded of the one remaining hour. He muttered to himself and then added audibly, "If she doesn't take next week, it's going to be too bad." He was quite deliberate in his painting and careful about his choice of colors. As he used the paper towels he announced: "This week I'm going to adopt a new person to get them for you and when he is through, he can get someone else." He wanted to be represented by a substitute after he left. He worked and talked, and when he was through he was very exacting in his requirements about how everything should be kept for his final hour. At the end of this hour he was more deliberate in his efforts to prolong his stay.

In his last hour, Jimmy looked around casually, and thought there was not much to do. In manner and word he indicated an easy readiness to be through with therapy. He gave many details about his new club made up of neighborhood kids. However, his regret at leaving focused in the question he raised about who would take his time and he expressed some irritation by saying he would like to smash the telephone.

He thought it would be nice to leave a record on the blackboard so he wrote May 31, which was his ending date. He gave elaborate instructions as to how the date was to be changed and how a record was to be kept of everyone who came into the therapist's office. Then he fixed the alarm clock to ring when his time was up but asked if he could have five extra minutes. The therapist quietly commented on how hard it was to end, and as he stood close to her, he agreed without any apology or exaggeration.

Toward the end of this final hour Jimmy said, "I've a good one to put down on the blackboard, write Dr. D. is nurts." He followed this with a few aggressive remarks and then wrote "I am nuts" and pinned the slip of paper on which this was written onto the front of the therapist's dress. In this final act he left behind with the therapist a quality of his former self which the word "nurts" partially described. When the alarm clock went off, which he had included in this extra time allowed him, he said good-by and with a warm smile joined his mother and left the clinic.

The mother, in her last appointment, described Jimmy as being "an easier boy to live with," and in this change she felt much closer to him. She described her own change too! "I no longer try to see everything from his point of view," indicating that she too was in possession of herself as a person in her own right, and as Jimmy's mother.

Some children maintain a constant connection with their outside activities in all that goes on in their therapeutic hours. The hours are full of talk about their problems, their family and activities. Other children come for a considerable series of interviews without much reference to what goes on beyond the walls of the therapist's office. It would be a mistake to conclude that there is greater therapeutic value in one or the other way children may use to verbally locate their problems. To reach that conclusion would mean that the emphasis of the therapist was placed on what the child says and does rather than on the child who is responding in one way or the other. In the two cases described in detail the contrast in the verbal content of the therapeutic interviews is striking. Solomon talked about his behavior in other situations, particularly at home, to express and clarify his feelings in his relationship with the therapist. Jimmy, on the other hand, rarely mentioned his outside activity and focused his conversation on the immediate things he was doing with the therapist. In both instances there was real growth during the course of therapy.

The important point for the therapist to be clear on is that children are able to use the therapeutic relationship in different ways to achieve important changes in themselves. The same is true of the different ways they can adopt to avoid any significant connection with the therapist. The therapy is in the use that the child makes of the experience and not merely in the verbal activity that focuses on one content or another.

From these cases a clearer understanding of the place of content can be obtained. Actually, it makes little difference what the verbal content is as long as the therapist maintains an orientation to the use the child is making of this, and of his interests and activity, verbal and muscular, in establishing his relationship with the therapist. Bearing this in mind the therapist can avoid the pitfalls of getting caught in trying to obtain a particular content where the emphasis shifts to *what* the child is saying and away from the child who is saying it.

8

FACTORS THAT INTERFERE
WITH THERAPY

BY THEIR behavior a parent and a child may indicate a need
for help. Some parents may be able to take the initiative in
seeking a better way of living together by coming to a specific source of help, such as a child guidance clinic. This
move, however, does not of necessity mean that either child
or parent can use the help that is available. Sometimes neither
one is really ready to do anything about the mutual difficulties. This chapter, therefore, will be devoted to a discussion of some of the influences that can interfere with therapy.

A fundamental thesis of this book is that change in a human
being, whether child or adult, cannot be brought about by
forces that operate purely externally to that person. The
word "change" refers to the inner reorganization of an individual around forces that impinge upon him and that are
an integral part of his living reality. The individual may
have had nothing to do with originating these influences and
they may be entirely beyond his control. But his responses
to them are his own adaptations to these realities and bring
the individual into an active relation to them. The external
influence may or may not be modified by these adaptations,
but the individual will have changed and thus a new configuration emerges.

A child guidance clinic is one external influence in the lives of parents and children before they seek the use of its services. A parent may have known of the clinic's existence and may have had some interest in the fact that such an organization was available for parents and children needing help. But it has no vital meaning for a particular parent and child until they seek to use these services for problems in their own lives. At that point the clinic ceases to be an external force and is linked to their lives through the feelings that are awakened by the step they have taken. Immediately it becomes a source of comfort or danger or sometimes both, a cure-all or just another "fad" or a place where parents anticipate finding solid values around which to effect changes in their living relationships with their children.

Whether or not the journey upon which a parent and child embark when they seek the help of the professional staff of a child guidance clinic is successful will depend upon many factors. Two immediately stand out. One concerns the skill and the point of view of the individuals on the staff who assume the responsibility of carrying out the therapeutic work which a parent and a child seek and need. The second concerns the readiness and capacity of the parent and child who are needing help to make effective use of these skills to bring about changes in themselves, and to give meaning to these changes in the continuing realities of their day-to-day living. We can see at once that these two significant, large factors are essential elements in the new configuration that emerges when one person reaches out for the help that another person can offer.

In this chapter I shall emphasize the influences that can interfere with the constructive results of the child-therapist relationship. This relationship is a new whole that is invested with great meaning. That is, in a measure, because it has both unity and integrity in itself; but even more important, it is a part of a larger whole, that is, of what a parent can accomplish through working with the social worker on his aspect of the problem, as well as what the child is accomplishing; and beyond but related to these two, what they are able to do in the concrete expressions of this in their everyday realities.

The therapist who loses sight of the wider implications of what he and the child are doing together may introduce an overwhelming barrier to therapy. There is danger of becoming so wrapped up in the particular experience that is going on between therapist and child that it gets insulated from other aspects of living. There is greater danger that this may happen when all therapeutic effort centers on the child. The inclusion of the parent in a therapeutic program is a recognition of the wider nature of the problem, and, in itself, may prevent the isolation of the therapeutic situation from the continuing experiences of the child's day-to-day living.

Effective therapy with a child depends upon the changes a child can make in himself through the medium of a therapeutic relationship. The therapist has no power to do that changing. If his point of view stems from a belief that he can change a child, irrespective of the participation of the child, he will introduce a real barrier to therapy. A therapist can participate in these changes only when he knows and feels his essential limitations. The child may start, as I have indicated previously, with the expectation that the therapist possesses this power to cure. He comes prepared to defend himself against this power, or to become its passive recipient who disowns his capacity to do anything about his difficulties. The therapist who assumes such a role will find himself blocked from the beginning, and will center the entire emphasis of his therapy on what is done to the child and not on what he can help the child to do. These general considerations emphasize the significance of a therapist's point of view, and the use he can make of his skill and understanding.

A therapist with children must start with a clear acceptance of the fact that a child can defeat any therapeutic skill he possesses. A child can hold himself aloof from establishing any relationship with a therapist, and, by doing that, allow nothing positive to get into this experience. If he continues to maintain the projection of all the curing force on the therapist, nothing will happen in the therapy and the child may end right where he begins.

The nature of the child's relationships in which, actually, his problem is rooted has considerable bearing on the course of therapy. How this becomes a determining factor will be illustrated through some actual case material. Neither child nor parent may be ready to effect a breaking up of the totality of their interlocked selves even though they describe in words the impossibility of continuing further the way they are living. The therapeutic process offers a first step toward this (if they are ready for it), and the coming to the clinic for help and beginning this together is concrete evidence of some readiness. Certainly their willingness to take a road leading to self-differentiation here receives a real test, particularly in a procedure that allows both parent and child to have an active part in all that happens. Whether they can continue with what they have initiated remains in every case an open question.

Sam, five years old, was the only child of a devoted and possessive mother who was the dominant emotional influence in the family. The father played a passive role and, according to the mother, was always co-operative with her and helped to maintain a family atmosphere of "sweetness" and "loveliness." The mother stressed that they never quarreled and told how they agreed on everything. Evidently there was room for little individual difference in the family picture she painted in this first interview.

Sam's difficulties centered mainly on eating. He would

not eat solid food, and on the infrequent occasions when the parents applied pressure to make him eat, he reacted with abdominal pains which brought prompt medical attention. The threat to vomit, which he could and frequently did carry out, effectively neutralized the mother's efforts to change his eating habits. Sam was in control, and the constant medical attention, including an "exploratory laparotomy," served only to tighten his grip on the family situation.

The picture of sweet reasonableness, however, was maintained in all the parent's efforts to bring about normal eating habits in this boy who was determined to maintain his infantile relationship with his mother. The fact that she could not or would not give any real expression of the way she felt about her futile efforts to make him take some responsibility was evidence of how much she was caught in this problem. In the face of all the difficulties and irritations, her constant request was, "Now, Sam, dear, will you eat?" and his constant response was, "Yes, mother dear, I would like to." To maintain this unreal relationship both had to respond with feelings that had no reality. As a result their relationship was devoid of growth-inducing stimuli.

In the mother's initial interview, which was her first attempt to break up this deadlock and seek a different kind of help, she came closer to facing her own hostile and resentful feeling about the control this boy exercised over her entire life. "He controls our whole living, we are weak beside him," was her description. In admitting this element in Sam's problem, she placed less emphasis on the physical causes of his "sickness" and touched more on the stubborn "cruel" strength in the child who was always "outwitting" her and defeating her futile efforts to do anything. As an instance she told of tying his hands to stop his finger biting, when, after an hour he had said: "Mother dear, you should have tied them tighter."

The mother brought the boy for a single appointment, and a few days later she telephoned the social worker who had begun work with her, telling of her decision not to continue with the arrangements she had made for treatment. The mother's inability to continue what she had begun in those two hours brings clearly before us how a parent can block any therapeutic effort in working with children. Obviously, she could not bear the pain of separating herself from the child nor move in the direction of becoming a person in her own right. At this point the mother was in control of any steps that might be taken to help the child. The only constructive thing that the social worker could do at that time was to help the mother to accept her own decision to wait. This case brings out so clearly that the need for help, even when the situation is quite desperate as it was in this family, is no valid indication that parent and child are ready to use help.

Two years later, when Sam was seven, the mother again sought help and came in to tell how the problem was just as bad, if not worse, as it had been two years earlier. She told of their futile efforts in this interval to get Sam to eat and how their doctor had tried everything to bring about different eating habits. She described, with a strong admixture of pride and guilt, how she had stopped his vomiting when, in a moment of anger (which was quite rare for her) she fed his vomitus back to him. It made her sick to do it, but he did not vomit after that. Around the change which seemed to have taken place in her, the mother was helped to accept her greater readiness for help, both for herself and the boy. She brought out, with more real conviction, that she had no life of her own because of Sam, and she now recognized her own inability to effect changes in him without help. Through seven years of effort, characterized mainly by "sweet reasonableness," she had been unable to define any essential differences between herself and her only child.

In the one interview with Sam when he was five years old, he entered at once into play activity that clearly revealed the nature of some of his difficulties. He showed no reaction to leaving his mother, because, in feeling, he really was not leaving her. This beginning reaction made this case quite different from that of Solomon whom we discussed in Chapter VI. Sam started playing with the toy animals and described them as refusing to eat when he called them. He said with considerable emphasis, "They are very bad, they won't do what I tell them. I am going to punish them." But in spite of the drastic measures he adopted to make them eat, the animals remained bad by refusing to eat. He dramatized his whole dilemma in that hour when he projected all his difficulties into the play medium. If the mother had been able to continue, that might have been a real beginning of therapy. The deep impression this one therapeutic hour made upon Sam was clearly revealed two and a half years later when, on returning to the same therapist, he recalled vividly the details of that experience and duplicated the same play drama.[1]

Sam's manner at the beginning of each hour that followed rarely varied. He would greet the therapist in his debonnaire manner saying: "How are you today," and he positively "oozed" sweetness as he tried to make each hour a social call. He was painfully polite and never made any new move, however slight, without asking permission. At every point he maintained a rigid control of any other feeling expression

[1] The question is raised frequently about the value of appointments for a young child when the spacing allows a week's interval. This boy, after two years, responded as if no time had elapsed at all. He picked up the thread of that previous hour as if it had been the day before. It was amazing and most enlightening to see that happen.

although at times his play indicated the turmoil going on inside of him. At no point was there any letting down of the barriers that maintained his relation with the therapist on a controlled and artificial basis. He summed up the goal of his determination when he said in his third hour: "I want to be a doctor. I don't like to be the sick one. I like to be the well one." The therapist responded: "Sam, I know it is hard for you to let me be the doctor and you the one who comes for help." He bristled at this and maintained: "You are not a doctor here," and insisted that he came only to play and to get a rest from his teacher at school.

In the early phase of therapy this amount of determination is not a barrier but a necessary step through which the child can discover both the value and the limitation of his own strength. Many children who start their therapeutic experience with this much determination begin to move toward a more constructive use of that strength when they find a person who can both respect and accept it without being controlled by it. In putting that much fight into a new experience a child becomes engaged in a relationship which allows both struggling and yielding. But Sam, who started with so much inner and outer control of all feeling, continued to maintain these unrelated, artificial expressions of himself. That was his basic problem. He could never risk any real feeling in any relationship, and, in consequence, he had no friends among children. A few adults seemed to like him for his "politeness" and the solicitude which he always expressed about their welfare.

Sam found it hard to admit that there was any reason for his coming to see the therapist. In the first few hours he dodged any discussion of why he came, or that he had any other than the most pleasant feelings about coming. In his fifth hour he was building what he called his secret house. It had only one door and he held the key. The therapist commented: "You want to hang on to that key, Sam." He replied: "Yes, and even if someone got it, it wouldn't help, as there is a secret way of unlocking the door." The therapist added that he was giving a clear picture of how he felt about coming, when he was so determined not to let the therapist really know him, and that we were not getting very far. He said, "No, we haven't and I don't think we will." Sam then launched into a war game, saying, "These soldiers think they are going to win but they can't. I am too tricky for them." When the therapist commented Sam could be too tricky for him, he immediately took the meaning of this away from the immediate situation and put it all on the play.

The play activity of children in therapy provides a natural medium for expressing feeling. This point was discussed in Chapter V and also, as in the case of George, in Chapter III. Play provides a natural language for the feeling of the child as he moves toward a more real and immediate use of feeling in his relationship with another. But with Sam play provided an effective escape from feeling. It was true that he came somewhat closer to real feeling through his play activity, but he was quite able to keep himself from going beyond a certain point.

If Sam had been able to share with the therapist any of his secrets, the important point would not have been the particular thing revealed, but his willingness and freedom to share. The therapist was not trying to elicit any particular content but was concerned with helping this boy to share some feeling about what he was doing. The secret house play brought out Sam's ambivalence. He wanted the therapist to find the way in because he was an unhappy youngster who wanted to change, but he wanted the therapist to do it all. Then Sam again could prove more openly his control, because of his ability to defeat any efforts to unlock the door.

Such doors are opened only when one respects their right to be closed.

In the fifth hour Sam came more into the open about the reasons for coming. He did it in a safe and characteristic way. He started by saying: "Can I ask you a question?" and before the therapist could say anything he added: "Doctor, I don't eat very well. Can you tell me why—now give me the answer." Thus he laid down the plan of his battle as he persisted in his demand that the doctor give the right answer. He reserved for himself the right to decide which answers were correct. When the comment was made that there were probably too many people trying to make him eat, he promptly said, "No, that's not the right answer." Sam persisted in his question and came closer to showing real anger when he could not draw the therapist into the trap of giving specific answers. But immediately again he diverted his anger into a war game with soldiers. When the comment was made about his being mad at not getting what he demanded, he blithely responded, "Only dogs get mad."

He started his seventh hour with this riddle, "If there is a man inside a house and there is no way of escaping, and there is a man outside of a house and there is no way of getting in, how does the man get out and how does the other man get in." The baffling thing about Sam was his ability to give such clear formulations of his whole life dilemma, and yet to do so little with that ability. The therapist related this riddle to the one he stated about his eating and said, " Sam, I don't have any ability or desire to make you do anything you don't want to do." He challenged what he was finding hard to accept, that the therapist did not have all the answers. "Why can't you? My mother and father can, or anyone I am closely related to can." The therapist expressed a doubt about Sam's being closely related to anyone as he seemed to have to do so much fighting, and with his sweet innocence he said, "I don't fight." In one sense Sam was right because his struggle against eating never seemed like actual fighting.

Underlying this whole picture there was a great deal of fear which never came through as fear. All feeling, whether positive or aggressive, was either dramatized in an artificial and unreal type of sweetness, or given a physical expression such as vomiting. It was easy to see the nature of the relationship everyone had with this boy. It could not be any more real than the feeling he put into it, a fact which is true of every relationship in life but uniquely true of the therapeutic relationship.

As interviews continued, Sam maintained his determined pressure to get an answer. "I am going to keep on asking until you give me the answer. I just want an answer." The therapist commented: "Sam, I think you are giving your own answer." He looked surprised and the therapist went on to comment that the answer was in his determination to get just what he wants, and to give little or nothing himself. "You may have to go on fighting because at the moment you don't want an answer, but it is clear you do want to fight to get one." He persisted in his effort as the therapist said directly he could not give him the answer. "Then I'll tell my mother and she will give it up." The therapist commented: "When you stop trying to make others do all the work or when they decide to give up, you may get around to trying to see what you yourself can do." He said, "I can't." And then in one of the rare, unguarded moments in this entire case, Sam said: "I can if I try." But he caught himself at once and added, "But I do try, can you give me the answer?"

It has been brought out in previous discussions that the act of a parent in bringing a child for help implies a dissatisfaction with the child's present behavior and the necessity for change. The child's determination not to be changed naturally is roused. But this should not be by the direct efforts of the therapist to bring about the changes desired. Sam's reactions were a constant challenge to get the therapist to take full responsibility for changing him. As a result, it was difficult to steer a course that helped him to struggle but that did not engage him in a struggle. Around his demand for an answer to "Why don't I eat," his struggle revolved. No answer would have had any value until he was ready to participate in finding the answer. If that had happened it would have been the beginning of a new and more responsible feeling about himself in relation to another person. It would have been a growth step away from the determined effort to maintain an infantile and undifferentiated feeling about himself. Several times the therapist commented about Sam's determined stand against growing up and toward staying three years old, an age he gave as the beginning of his difficulty. Rather plaintively he said: "That wouldn't do me any good; even if I wanted to I wouldn't get anywhere if I were still a baby."

Through this period Sam had periods when his exaggerated eating difficulties would completely disappear. But no real change underlay this. He would eat better to gain a temporary end. Just before his birthday he quickly ate everything that was offered him. He wanted a particular present, and once he had it, all the eating difficulties returned. There was the same control in his eating better as there had been in his refusing food.

The mother was able to get on a somewhat more real basis with him. This mother, who had always tried to make everything sweet and lovely and whose reaction to the most exasperating behavior was, "Now, Sam dear," could now begin to let her feeling come out for what it was. Her life had been one of "sacrifice," and it was a big event when she let herself go off on a week-end trip and leave the boy. She was beginning to assume the role of a mother and could react with her real feeling and not with the false sweetness that veiled any real expression of feeling. The boy's sickness had held her in a vise. Through the determined use of his symptoms he became much stronger than the mother, who had clung in the futile position of trying to make him eat.

It became increasingly apparent that Sam was using his problem to perpetuate the same kind of relationship with his therapist. This was clear in his tenth hour. There was more open recognition of the battle he was putting up against taking any responsibility for himself. Sam asked: "Can't you help me win this battle?" I told him I could if he really would let me help. "Then give me an answer." "Sam, that wouldn't be winning because you would have to fight me on any answer I gave. The battle you can win is in coming out of that secret house you have built around yourself." Then the therapist repeated an earlier comment he had made about too many people trying to make him eat and added: "Sam, I am not interested in how you eat or when you eat. I am interested in helping you to be clear on what you are ready to do about your eating habits. Maybe you are not ready to do anything different." Sam was close at this point to showing some real anxiety and violently began ringing a bell, in the role of a vendor, to cover up his disturbed feeling. The therapist asked him what he was selling and Sam replied, "This room." The therapist suggested he was finding it hard to go on when he was not getting his own way. Sam wanted to know if he was coming the following week, and here the therapist fell into the trap saying, "Yes, and you will be coming until you and I can get some of your difficulties straightened out." Instantly he responded: "Then I'll try to make it take a long time." His eating problem was his means of perpetuating an infantile relation to his mother, and now he was trying to make it the basis of maintaining this relationship with the therapist. For him to begin assuming any responsibility for his problem in this potentially growth-inducing experience meant the first step in ending the infantile mode of living to which he was so determined to cling. It would also have meant the first step in ending his relationship with the therapist.

Sam found it hard to accept any limitation to his unreal sense of power. This came out in some of the play activity which revealed much turmoil that he could not or would not admit. He was fussing with some clay, and said: "I'm going to make something that I can't make, and I will keep at it if it's the last thing I do." When the therapist commented, "You don't like to think anything is too hard," he announced, "I can do anything I want to do." This was a challenge and when it was not accepted Sam said meekly and with more realness, "But I can't." Then he announced his desire to own the building and "you with it." The therapist added: "Then you could make me do anything you wanted." He thought that would be perfect. But around the further comment, "Sam, you become quite scared when you meet someone who cannot be controlled," he said, "I guess you are right—in some little way." This was quite a concession. He went back, however, to his clay and started beating it vigorously, saying, "Bad pieces of clay. It didn't do what I wanted it to do." He started hammering vigorously on a piece of wood and finally split it. He announced with a triumphant look, "It gave up," and the therapist remarked, "It is easier to manage the wood than yourself," and commented on the anxiety Sam has around giving up the struggle that was preventing him from growing up. He responded by getting a bigger piece of wood and saying, "I never give up." It was hard to believe that a seven-year-old child could maintain such a powerful front against any of the yieldings which living and growing con-

stantly required. The totality of all his responses invested
yielding also with that same complete quality. To yield
meant a total loss of self, with the ensuing fear which con-
tinually activated the determination so in evidence in each
minute of his hour with the therapist.

In his eleventh hour Sam announced that he had another
week of perfectly normal behavior, and told about it with
the same purpose of forcing an answer from the therapist.
He prefaced his announcement by asking: "I have a question,
will you answer it?" He was encouraged to find out for himself. Then he told of being "good" all week and, "On Sunday
I went to see Snow White and immediately after the show
I was bad again. Now why did I?" The therapist asked what
the picture had to do with it and he said, "I wanted to see it."
The therapist was quite direct in his comment and said:
"Sam, you are always looking for an answer from somebody
else to explain your goodness and your badness. You knew
the only way of seeing that picture was by promising to be
good." Instantly he made the significant reply, "No, not by
promising to be good, but by being good." The therapist
smiled and said, "The strain was too great, being good lasted
only as long as you wanted it to last." He looked at the therapist and said, "You're right—this much," and measured off
a half inch with his fingers.

In the thirteenth hour the therapist helped him to bring
the struggle more into the open and asked: "Sam, why do you
come to see me?" He tried to turn that back and said: "You
know why I come. Why do I come?" The therapist persisted
and added: "That is what I am asking." Sam added: "I come
because my mother takes me. I don't know why I come."
"Sam, do you really think you can fool me on that?" "On
what?" he parried, as he tried to end the direct discussion initiated by the therapist. He turned the discussion to one aspect

of his therapeutic relationship he could not control when he asked: "Can I come here anytime?" The therapist replied: "No Sam, and that has always bothered you, because you come at a time which I set, and you have to leave when I say your time is up." He had maintained from the beginning that the therapist had sent for him, and he had some justification for this belief because the mother had told him before the first visit that the doctor had wanted to see him. This was a hurdle that was hard to clear, and the boy made effective and determined use of it. In the discussion of this hour he used it to avoid any expression of his own desire to come to the clinic. The therapist went on with the discussion and said: "I assume, Sam, that in coming to see me you come for a little help." "I do," and he added: "I want to know why I don't eat." The therapist responded: "Sam, you can't answer that alone, nor can I. It is a question we have to work on together, but I do not know if you want to help in that way." In his meekest and sweetest manner, which had no realness in it at all, he replied: "But I do want help. I want to do something." That desire did not get beyond his lips.

In this hour he commented about the therapist's taking notes and immediately tried to make this a reasonable thing about which he would admit no feeling. But the hour had stirred him considerably and an unusual thing for him happened. He was playing with the soldiers, and suddenly he picked one up and threw it, with a momentary flash of anger. It was over in a flash but it was the only time he ever let his guard down and allowed a spontaneous burst of anger. The therapist said: "Sam, I know you feel that way inside but it is hard to let me see it." Quickly he regained control and sweetly said, "Oh no—is that a good answer?"

Through these hours the therapist stressed Sam's continued evasion of any real responsibility for his own feeling and his own part in the helping process. Usually he sparred or played dumb as he said, "You know I'm not very smart." But it became clearer that he was not going to make headway toward finding a different balance in himself. There were several aspects of his relationship with the therapist that disturbed him: the note taking, the therapist's smoking (he had been told that he was allergic to tobacco and that no one was to smoke in his presence, thus putting another weapon in his hands), the other children who came, the regularity of his time for coming, his inability to win at checkers, and so on. Sam would protest about each of these, then brush aside all the feeling that they roused. He agreed that he did feel angry at times, and when the therapist said he found it hard to let any of that feeling come into the open he replied, "I never will," and usually ended his statement with "Only dogs get mad."

His play activity was scattered and usually without a goal or purpose. When he started to paint, it ended in smearing. When he began to write on the blackboard he finished with a lot of scratches. There were a few exceptions and usually these brought him closer to significant aspects of his difficulty. One day he described a painting he was making as the bottom of the sea, and there was a pot of gold down there that he wanted to get. "What would you do with it Sam?" "I would eat it," he replied. The therapist said that only in that way could he be sure it belonged to him. He quickly said, "I don't want to be rich. If I had a lot of money the bandits might come and take it away." This was such a clear statement of the constant fear he had that someone, in this instance the therapist, was trying to take away what he owned. He could go no further with this. His eating was always invested with the determination to own, in a complete way, all that he took in. But to use and live with what he owned seemed to mean its loss. He had to own a thing completely or not at all. That was the pattern of living which constituted the life problem which he could not break up in his therapeutic relation.

The ending was initiated by the therapist. After five months of weekly appointments it was clear there was a stalemate. At first Sam couldn't admit any of his own feeling about ending and lamely said, "My mother will be glad." He was told he would have three more appointments and he said with more feeling than usual, "Won't I ever be coming again?" and was told that would depend on whether he felt he needed to come. With more realness than usual he replied, "I like to come but I don't know why—I hope I need to come."

The ending did stir this amazing boy into something that was different, but this was elusive and hard to define. In the next to the last hour he brought up his eating difficulties. Sam made some clay doughnuts and asked, "Would you die if you ate them?" Following this question he was closer to bringing out some of the fear that eating held for him. To eat was to grow and to grow meant that he would eventually die. He wanted to grow but not by his own efforts. He brought this out by lying on the floor and pretending to be asleep. Quickly he jumped up and said, "Look, I've become a man. I've changed myself forever, and I can prove it. I don't play with those baby toys, isn't that enough proof?" The therapist doubted if it was enough, so he repeated the performance in order to change more. Then he said, "We are both men," then changed that to, "You are a child. I am a man." He could not face his own difference which the termination of the interviews forced him to face. He had set his determination against any breaking up of the fixed pattern he had held to with such tenacity. It was in keeping with this pattern that he ended by making the therapist the little one and retained his own unreal feeling of power which he could not use for his own growth. "You are so little and I am so big—in thirty years you'll grow up and be little," were his ending remarks.

Three years later the therapist saw this boy in a hospital bed where he had been placed because of "abdominal pain." He was cheerful and healthy in appearance and free from pain. The boy did not recognize the therapist which was not surprising in view of the fact he never did establish a relationship with him. It was an interesting contrast to the vivid and minute recall of his first interview after the two-year lapse. That first interview touched a quality that struck deep. The other interviews touched only the unreal and left no mark. Evidently he had regained complete control of both family and doctor and they were continuing to respond to his every pain. Why should he want to grow up and give up the neurotic pattern of living which enabled him to deny any responsibility for himself?

He was able to maintain amazing control over all emotional responses during the five months period of weekly interviews. Only around ending was he able to allow the therapist to have a fleeting contact with a quality in him that seemed more real. He was able to maintain, through his bland and unreal sweetness, a position that took in little and gave up nothing. He seemed incapable of having any real feeling. Rarely did he show evidence of anxiety, he never got angry, with the exception of the momentary flash, and he always maintained the sugary politeness which kept his therapist right where he was determined to keep him. He was never really good and never really bad. He was an artifact.

There can be no therapy with a child who cannot or will not experience real feeling. There can be no relationship without the more alive and responsible evidences of a self which are involved in the expression of feeling. The artificial and dramatized substitutes such as were described in this case allowed none of the connections essential for growth and therapy. It is equally true there can be no therapy when the therapist assumes an impassive role and allows little evidence of being a human being himself, as the other participant in the relationship. The therapist who tries too hard to maintain an "objective attitude" may become an automaton in a relationship with a child who needs the unobtrusive warmth of a friendly human being who possesses the skill and strength to help him come to grips with his emotional turmoil. Friendliness alone cannot help the child, nor can skill of itself be therapeutic. But when these two are combined in the person of the therapist, a setting is created that offers a more favorable medium for the child to find himself. Without the human element in the therapist, the child who needs a great deal may be thrown back into himself and be one step further away from a healthier connection with reality.

It is possible for a therapist to block therapy by trying to be too good and understanding. An aggressive, fighting child who has been running roughshod over every limit and every person will find more anxiety roused by the therapist who is too giving and understanding on the theory that the child needs to be "loved" because of "affect-deprivations." In the first place there is no genuine love in such an attitude on the part of a therapist. Instead this attitude comes closer to being a form of "seduction" that requires the child to love in return. It is a false situation and a child is quick to detect the falsity and to proceed to defeat the unnatural sweetness by continuing to be a child no one can love. The anxiety of being trapped stirs more aggression. Such a child craves a strong person able to allow freedom of feeling and limitation of the action. A failure to understand the constructive value of limits with such a child will result in a failure to see and touch the living child behind the aggressive front, the child who is fearful of his own positive, gentle quality. A deprived child who covers up his need for affection by an air of bravado and attack cannot make any connection with a therapist who is so aware of the child's affectional needs that he fails to provide the necessary control to the child's aggression. A therapist who can only provide such a child with "gentle understanding" forces that child to set all the limits himself, and he cannot do that. He needs a therapist who can be sufficiently real to provide the necessary controls, while at the same time he can strengthen the child's capacity to express the positive feelings which underly his aggressive action. Just being good and gentle with such a child will introduce a barrier that may push the child away from the therapist.

Frequent mention has been made of the blocking effects of the therapist's over-great zeal to cure, and little more need be said of that here. In summarizing some of the forces that can block therapy, this particularly stands out. The desire of the therapist to provide help, of itself, never can be therapeutic. He may have the necessary skill and an understanding of the causal factors that have created behavior disturbances and still be powerless to effect a change in a patient. The patient's use of this skill is the essential part of the therapeutic influence. There is intention to help implied when one assumes the responsibility of the therapist's role. That is both inevitable and necessary. It is the more purposeful emphasis of this intention that prevents the child from participating in his own change. A skillful therapist will know that the child comes with the expectation of being changed and will help him respond either for or against this expectancy, depending upon how he feels. But when a child meets a person who immediately starts to "train" him in patterns of behavior that are foreign to him at that time, the child is left with no alternative other than yielding to or fighting against the "synthetic" purposes of the therapist. The essential element of differentiation, which is inherent in therapy, is put to one side by this too intentional desire to treat.

Without differentiation there can be no growth. Living can never be the total thing which Sam tried to make of it, and retain any element of normality. The very essence of normality in living relationships springs from the reality of difference which is the product of differentiation. In therapy, the same principles hold true, and the child who fights against being a real person in his own right and maintains, as Sam did, a position that accepts responsibility for little or nothing will be able to defeat any therapeutic effort. When there is the inability to give anything up, then there can be no sharing or creative use of the individual's difference, which comes only through growth and separation.

When the other half of this book is written, the half that deals with the parents' participation in the therapeutic process, other factors will have to be considered which either accelerate or interfere with a successful outcome to what parents initiate when they bring their child for help. Their readiness for a new orientation to themselves and their children meets a living test in the part they assume in therapy. Can they bear the separations that are required, not only by the therapeutic process but by the demands of their everyday reality; can they allow a child to have a real part in the solution of his problem, and break up the more complete responsibility they have taken for the problem, and the child? Can they assume responsibility for the part of the problem that belongs to them and work on it in their relationship with a social case worker? How can the skill and function of the social case worker, working with the parent, be defined in a clinic setup so as to enable the parent to work on this area of his life without spreading that over his entire adult life? These are some of the questions that differentiate therapy from case work and need a full book for their discussion. But the way they are answered in the actual work with a parent determines in no small way the difference between success and failure in a therapeutic effort that involves both parent and child.

As I have said before, the importance of the therapeutic experience stems from the fact that it occurs in relation to the more total living experiences of the individual being helped. It does not occur in isolation. The therapist can become for a child a symbol of the new he may be finding, not just in the therapeutic hour but at the same time in his school, on the street with the other children, and in the home. The therapist must maintain a broad orientation, as otherwise he may become a symbol of a too narrowed life and one in which the child finds no connection to the continuing realities of his life. The ending phase which we are now ready to discuss will be a constructive phase or one destructive of the values gained in the therapeutic hour in direct proportion to the meaning of the experience in the realities out and beyond the walls of the clinic in which the child has found a source of help to start him on his way.

9

THE ENDING PHASE OF THERAPY

THE VALUES of the therapeutic experience in which a child
and therapist are engaged emerge in part around the fact that
this relationship is begun with the goal of its eventual termination. From the first hour this is the basic orientation of the
therapist. Each move the therapist makes that helps the child
to be a participant in his own change is one that helps that
child to assume responsibility for a self which he can accept
as uniquely his, and which is the very core of his living. With
this orientation, the ending phase of therapy becomes a process of affirming or reaffirming the difference a child perceives in himself as he develops within the steady framework
of a relationship made possible by a therapist and child together.

From the outset the therapist has no desire other than to
use his relationship to assist the child to be free finally of the
need for this specialized help. The child's feelings are at the
center of the experience, and the therapist is in a position to
encourage the child to use him in whatever ways he can to
grow toward a clearer awareness and acceptance of his own
child's self with all that is involved in living with parents,
siblings, and companions. The child may use the therapist to
symbolize the good or bad parent, the benevolent or the
tyrannical despot, or the possessor of magic to cure. These
shifting roles, which the child assigns to the therapist, who

holds steadily to his real role, spring from the heart of the child's turmoil, and represent his efforts to find a solution for his difficulties. The therapist does not need the child to satisfy his own needs and, in the midst of the changing demands of the child, is able to maintain his own integrity. The therapist who is free to be himself [1] can respond to the child's feelings in terms of their meaning to the child. Then he can be ready to assist the child through the differentiating steps of therapy which lead gradually into and through the ending phase, the essence of which is the child's affirmation of himself as an individual, not in isolation but in relation to others.

When the emphasis is placed on the word "ending" it is necessary to keep in mind that this is not a one-sided concept. Actually it describes only half of a life process. Designating the final culmination scene of an educational experience as "commencement day" is not the incongruity it has seemed to many people. This phrase incorporates the positive aspects that belong to every ending experience. The emphasis is not merely on the ending of something already past, but on the new which is being ushered in. The leaving of the old and the beginning of the new constitute the ever-recurring shifting of the scenes in human development. The old is terminated with full regard for the values and satisfactions that have accrued from it. If these values must, however, be measured and felt only in the circumstances in which they were experienced originally, then they cease to be growth-inducing influences and lose their positive meaning. Values from any life experience retain their positive meaning only as the

---

[1] I want to emphasize again that this statement implies a human quality of warmth and understanding that invests the professionally disciplined maturity of a therapist with a quality a child or adult can feel related to. A ten-year-old boy in constant conflict with authority came for his first hour evidently expecting a heavy handed disciplinarian. After his first, he described his puzzle about this person by saying: "That man is a little touched but I like that guy." This boy couldn't quite understand this new person but he knew how he felt about him.

individual is free to use them in the ever-recurring newness of living. This is not forgetting and repressing the old, but it is using the old to provide the structure of the new. Thus, there is the continuum so essential, not only for individuals, but for the cultures in which they move and live.

An essential quality of the neurotic individual is his inability to be free from a past he will not or cannot part with. When an individual is rooted in a "past present" and fears to loosen the anchorage to which he clings, he will not be able to use the satisfactions which he can legitimately carry over from the past to give meaning to the new. The new becomes a threat to be avoided. The neurotic is the person who has difficulty in ending any phase of living and constantly has his vision fastened on a past [2] that can neither be recaptured nor relinquished. This is the intolerable life dilemma described so vividly by Matthew Arnold in the individual "wandering between two worlds—the one dead, the other powerless to be born." [3]

A typical life situation of parent and child presented to a child guidance clinic is one in which parent and child are mired in a relationship which no longer works, but which neither one has the power to end. Such individuals are held together by an apparently insoluble struggle which must find some solution if the individuals involved are to gain any separate sense of their own values. A fifteen-year-old girl described the dilemma of this deadlock when she said: "My mother and I are closer to each other when we quarrel; otherwise we don't have anything to say." In the everyday life about us we constantly see individuals trying to effect these

[2] A facetious description of the "woofus bird" as one who has eyes in the back of his head to see where he came from because he does not like to see where he is going is a good description of neurotic behavior.

[3] From the stanzas of the Grande Chartreuse in "Poems of Matthew Arnold, 1840–1866" (J. M. Dent and Sons, London, and E. P. Dutton & Co., New York), p. 258.

separations in behavior patterns incompatible with healthy development. The escape into sickness, the explosive running away of the child and adolescent, the breaking up of families through its members' failure to find harmonious ways of being individuals within the family group are extremes to which individuals go in their efforts to destroy and escape from the deadlocks that occur in human relationships.

When a parent makes a move to seek the help a therapist and case worker can offer for a problem in his child, he is taking a step away from clinging to the untenable past in his relationship with a child, and toward finding a better way of living with the child. The therapist enters this picture at the point where a parent and child may be reaching out toward ending this long-standing struggle. When viewed in this way, the entire therapeutic experience is one of ending, and becomes symbolic of the new for which a parent and child are reaching. In itself a new experience it, too, will have its own ending and become another past. This is achieved around the affirmation of the new qualities which gradually came into being through therapy, but which remain when the therapeutic relationship itself is relinquished. It is this emphasis which helps us to understand the ending phase as a process, and an integral part of the whole therapeutic experience.

Ending is, as I have said, an integral part of the growth process initiated in the first hours of a therapeutic experience. In order that this phase of therapy shall acquire its full meaning for the child it must be brought into relation with a plan that gives clearer definition of what the child is ready to do. When the child has reached a point where both he and the therapist are aware of his readiness to bring their relationship to a close, a plan for effecting this is discussed between them. The child is helped to be an active participant in making the plan. There are no clear-cut signals for a therapist to follow in knowing when a child is ready to make such a plan. The best guides are those supplied by the child, and are recognizable if the therapist maintains an orientation to the whole growth experience, and remains sensitive to the changes he has helped the child to bring about.

The changes in the feeling-tone of the hour, the changes in the verbal content, the changes a parent and child describe in their day-to-day relationship, the dream material which children bring, all these and others have great meaning not as isolated bits of behavior, but as parts that fit into a new whole which the child is helping to bring about. These responses become the indicators of the child's readiness to end, indicators which the therapist, sensitive to their meaning, can recognize and bring into the open.

Since therapy terminates as a new separation experience, the child needs opportunity to live through some of the conflicting feelings which are aroused by this step. The relationship to the therapist has come to have great meaning to the child. For many children this has been the means of gaining a new perspective about themselves and their relationships to others. When the ending phase approaches, the child feels he is leaving behind an important support and that he may be risking loss of what he has gained. There is anxiety in this separation just as there was anxiety in the separations at the beginning. The child needed a period of time in the beginning to find what he could be in this new relationship. And, in the ending phase, he will need to have a planned period in order to learn the meaning of this anxiety that is aroused by the prospect of assuming fuller responsibility for the changes he has effected through the help of the therapist.

The ending plan grows from the child's readiness to participate in making that plan. It becomes the more open and organized recognition by child and therapist of the progress made thus far. In the interviews given here, which lead up to the final hour of treatment, the child has opportunity to experience what it means, in feeling, to end a significant phase of living. The parent takes an active part in making an ending plan, and in their living through the final series of interviews, many reactions appear which give evidence of the fact that this is a stirring period for both child and parent. Some children swing from such extremes as wanting to come a thousand more times to asserting, "This is my last time." The first extreme represents the determination never to end, and the other swing of the pendulum indicates the child's determination to end entirely on his own terms and thus to avoid the anxieties that are necessarily awakened.

The plan of ending upon which the child and therapist agree now becomes a positive affirmation of the child's readiness to affirm the new in himself. The interviews that follow permit fuller expression of both the satisfactions and the anxieties and struggles the child feels around a plan he has helped to make. The mistake that was made with Jimmy (Chapter VII), in the ending phase of his therapy, lay in the failure of the therapist to sense, sufficiently early, the boy's readiness to end. Jimmy was ready to make a plan about six interviews before the final hour. When the therapist did not act at that time the struggle became focused on the making of the plan; that is, whether Jimmy should come two or four more times. The ending could have been more positive and constructive had the inevitable turmoil of ending grown from a plan of termination which Jimmy was ready to make without struggle, as really representing what he wanted and was ready to carry out.

Around ending the child may and frequently does experience anew some of the disturbance that characterized the beginning. This was clearly indicated in the two cases discussed in Chapters VI and VII. Some of the symptoms which have disappeared during the course of the therapeutic process may temporarily reappear as the child begins to assume responsibility for ending. These reactions of the ending phase frequently are mistaken as evidence that the child needs more help, rather than as partial efforts of the child to cling to a source of help which, in reality, he no longer needs or wants. To postpone the ending and fail to sense the meaning of these responses is a major error which may jeopardize the values that have emerged in the therapy by forcing the child to end negatively.

The child who can say, in his final hours of therapy, "I don't want to stop coming," yet can go ahead with his plans to end the treatment is giving to his feelings the partial expression so essential in normal living. This represents a constructive ending experience since the child is not using one feeling to deny another; instead both exist simultaneously, as partial expressions of feeling. It is the total withholding of a feeling expression in an individual that enables him to maintain an isolation that prevents the therapist from gaining any significant connection with him. The same totality of a possessively positive reaction can enable the child to avoid the dangers of separate and responsible living by trying to hold to the therapist as a symbol of his undifferentiated self. The child who in the course of therapy has found he can be a person in himself and have, at the same time, a relation with another, has broken up this unreal totality. Such a child is ready to end. He has found that he can be a whole in himself and still be a part of a larger whole. These partial feeling expressions in the ending phase become important indicators of this movement, and bring out the extent of the child's differentiation. Ending the old and beginning the new stand in natural relation to each other. The child can act on his impulse to live, which the ending of therapy represents in its creative meaning. However, associated with this impulse is some reluctance to let the old die. It is the balance between these aspects of feeling which is a part of each life experience in which the old and the new meet. The child may find this balance for the first time in this particular ending experience he has with his therapist.

Ending, therefore, does arouse some anxiety in children. The therapeutic relationship has come to have great meaning for a child and it would be unreal for the ending to be accomplished without any feeling. The important support the child needs from the therapist is help to express the feeling [4] that is awakened and not to have these responses interpreted as his need for further treatment. Such an interpretation of these responses would be like investing the original symptom with the control it had had previously and a vicious cycle would be established. If the anxiety aroused in ending is accepted as the evidence of the child's needing more help, this being held for further treatment rouses the child's real anxiety at feeling trapped in a relationship which the therapist cannot or will not help him to end. This vicious cycle more frequently occurs in adult therapy, or in child therapy which goes on without the participation of a parent.

The final phase of a therapeutic growth experience presents the therapist with a real test of his convictions and philosophy. The therapist knows that his relation to a patient is an important episode in that person's life, but that it is not, nor should it be, all of the patient's life. Thus the therapist's major interest from the beginning must be in helping the patient eventually to finish with this particular episode in his life. Only in that way can this unique relationship have any value. If a therapist adopts a protective role by trying to be-

---

[4] For a poignant example of the value of helping a child give outward expression to feeling see "Journey for Margaret" by W. S. White as condensed in the *Reader's Digest*, November, 1941. This child gained a relation to the new when she was helped to give vent to the surge of feeling aroused by the forceful separation from the old.

come a parent substitute in order to make sure before he "lets him go" that the patient will have no further difficulties, he cannot help the child to end. No therapeutic experience can provide a patient with a paid-up insurance policy against future difficulties although the anxiety centering about ending may activate the patient's need to have such assurance. This may be and frequently is a natural part of the ending process. The therapist can meet it, however, in a way that allows it to be a part and not the whole it becomes where the orientation is focused only on the anxiety. In that case treatment would go on and on.

The freedom the therapist has to help a patient end carries with it the patient's freedom to return if the future brings the need and desire for further help. When ending is understood as a process it does not have to carry the finality which the patient's anxiety may give it. Around ending many children bring up the question of a future visit. It is important for the therapist to let the child know he would be glad to have him come back to tell or show the therapist how he is getting along. Frequently children never act on this, but it is the immediate feeling that they can be free to act on it in the future which gives the necessary support which enables them to end. It is quite common to have a child come back after a lapse of time to prove to himself he is really through.[5] A single visit may be all that is necessary.

That this most important emphasis in ending, viz., that ending is a gradual process and not merely the date of the final appointment, may be better understood, the movement of an eight-year-old girl will be traced from the beginning to her final interview. In this sense, ending is understood as

[5] Recently a boy who ended treatment nearly ten years ago called his therapist on the telephone and recalled a number of incidents that happened when he was coming for help, and then said: "I just wanted to tell you I was getting along fine and thought you might like to know."

starting actually in the early phases of treatment, with the first awakenings of the separate self which the child discovers.

Grace, an eight-year-old girl, was as selfless a person as ever came to the clinic. Everything about her was wrong, and her nickname of "stink pants" called attention to the ever-present odor from constant enuresis. Grace's school work led her teachers to believe she was a defective child. The family was large and economically dependent. Yet in the family there existed a primitive type of unity. In their own crude way these parents were concerned with this girl who seemed to have so little. She received little attention, however, beyond nagging efforts to correct her diurnal and nocturnal enuresis. In the first interviews that the therapist had with Grace the child was able to do almost nothing. She did not seem to be particularly frightened nor was she antagonistic in any way. She had a selfless quality as if she had so little awareness of being anyone. Grace was unable to respond with any feeling until the end of the first hour when she said, in a barely audible tone of voice, that she wanted to return. The quiet and unobtrusive friendliness of the therapist, who could accept her as she was, helped Grace to smile a little as she left. Her solemn, distant quality continued through her second hour but at the end Grace expressed a desire to save a crude drawing she had made which portrayed, in form and description, a mixture of a boy and girl. While the making of this picture was a considerable step for Grace to take, it revealed again the uncertain selfless quality which she could not designate as either masculine or feminine. But she was gradually waking up to a feeling that she was somebody in this new relationship.

In the third hour, the awakening process was accelerated. Grace drew her chair closer and talked about her activity that had more purpose. She thought the tea set on the therapist's shelf was very dirty, and she washed all the pieces saying reprovingly, "You ought to be ashamed to have such dirty dishes." She had found the first medium upon which to project her feeling about herself and became the cleansing, critical person.

The quiet and forceful determination in this child was revealed in a remark she made about being left-handed. "The teacher told me to put the pencil in my right hand. I does it but I say no to myself." Her first movement toward a positive relationship was in finding a person who was not trying to make her over and who was helping her to give some outward expression to her negative feelings.

By the end of her fifth hour, Grace was an alive and alert little girl, rather impish in her manner but with a gaiety totally new for her. About this time she stopped her persistent soiling. She introduced two dolls into her play. She dressed the big one, handed it to the therapist and said, "This big one is yours, the small one is mine." She stood very close as she spoke of herself as the mother and the therapist as the father of these two girls. Grace was discovering she had a role in this relation to another person. It seemed clear to the therapist that the child she represented her doll to be was the newly emerging feeling she was gaining about herself. She was going through a psychological birth experience. Beginning with so little, she was becoming somebody.

The play activity in her seventh hour gave further evidence of her growth through this experience. She made a crude clay figure saying, "This is you." An identical figure was made and described as, "This is me." Then she put them together and said, "They are both you, they wear the same pants, you and me sleep, we will be together." Then she said "Half is me." A communal head was made for the two figures and then she was not in the figures at all. The therapist commented about her being a little anxious at being lost but

she replied, "No, I know you now and I'm not scared at all."
She did become a little anxious as she started to make herself
in another clay figure which indicated she was not yet ready
to assume a separate identity in the close and undifferentiated
relationship she had established.

When therapy is viewed as growth, the meaning of this
activity becomes clear as crystal. Grace had found a self in
this experience and felt closely related to the therapist who, at
the time, stood as the source of this new feeling about herself. She perceived a new security in this sense of belonging
but this aroused a new anxiety over the natural separation of
herself from this new source of life. She had dramatized in
the play of this one hour her progress to this point. She expressed little apprehension over the phantasied loss of her
identity because, in reality, she did not lose herself. She could
not have initiated this play activity until she made some progress toward acquiring some real feeling that she was a person
in her own right. She had accomplished this in the period preceding this hour.

Here is where the ending process began. In fact it began
when the child indicated in her play the growing evidence of
her difference from the therapist. Her movement in subsequent hours centered around being a person, separate and
different from the therapist. In the hour that followed, the
clay figures were there but she announced: "I am not going
to play with that today." She modeled clay into a baby, gave
it to the therapist saying, "This is your baby, it's a little girl."
Then she drew a house with a bedroom and had the therapist
in bed. "You are lazy," she said, and in the drawing she had
him falling out of bed, "Just as I did." The therapist was
wrong when he commented, "That's because you're a part of
me." Impatiently she corrected him and said: "No, here I
am," and drew a bed that was hers, separate and apart from
the other bed, in which she placed the therapist. The dif-

ferentiating step that had awakened anxiety a week earlier was now taken with assertion and confidence.

In the hours that followed Grace's play was easy and natural. The laughter and excitement were a part of the release she was finding in living. Once she commented: "You look like an old man sitting in that chair." Grace talked of her home and casually spoke of the time "when I used to wet myself." In her play and games the emphasis was on being the stronger and she tried to be a little tyrant in her bossiness. All this was a part of Grace's need to live and to test her new-found strength within the framework of this situation in which she found the first creative use of herself. More and more her interest shifted to home and school affairs, and events outside the room interested her more than things inside. She was indicating in both the verbal and feeling content of her hours, the extent of her progress and her readiness to end.

In her final hour, Grace brought two cents, asking, "Would you give these back if I gave them to you?" "What do you think I should do?" the therapist asked. Promptly Grace settled the question and said: "If I give them to you, I wouldn't have anything left—I'll keep them." This was the point at which she had arrived about herself, and shortly after this Grace made her own decision about ending which she carried through. Grace's mother was able to give the necessary support to this new child of hers. Through the mother's own participation, she found she could now really be mother to this child and not merely the corrector of her bad habits.[6]

In ending Grace's interviews, no plan was made in advance and as a result she had to take the whole responsibility of making her nineteenth hour the final one. A plan to end

---

[6] About once a year, this mother appears with Grace to show her off. She has become an interesting, normal child.

could have been made about five interviews earlier, as she was telling the therapist in several different ways that she was nearly through. He was a young therapist who did not sense fully what was going on, and he did not keep in sufficiently close contact with the social worker who was seeing the mother. The mother, however, worked toward an ending plan, and with that help, the child was able to come to her final hour and end without much difficulty. A much better ending would have ensued, however, if Grace could have had four or five interviews following the settling of a definite time when she would be through.

Through the medium of dream material, a therapist may gain his first awareness of the point at which a child is in the ending process. A most neurotic girl of thirteen whose theme song throughout life had been, "I was born too soon," devoted much of her energy to recapturing previous periods of life which had never provided growth-inducing satisfactions, particularly in infancy. She tried to exact from each new period in her life the satisfactions that belonged to, but were never obtained in, earlier periods. In a long period of therapy she had gained a much clearer perception of the values of being thirteen years old. Consciously she made many efforts to deny her improvement but she was more nearly ready to end than she could admit. About this time she told of a dream in which she went to a railroad station, accompanied by the therapist and by a child whom she identified as one she had met in the clinic waiting room. She was taking a journey with the other child (two parts of herself) and the therapist was at the station to see them off. It was a happy dream and she told it with a gaiety unusual in this sober and suspicious girl. It was a dream of movement and portrayed what she had been going through in her therapeutic relationship. In the discussion that followed, she denied its ending implications and asserted, "I'm not ready to leave," to which the therapist agreed. But in agreeing, the therapist helped her to accept that she was getting ready to leave and a plan was made that set the ending in two months.

In the period that followed she went through considerable turmoil. She vacillated between an angry mood in which she blamed the therapist for putting her out and a friendly mood in which she was more accepting of the changes in herself. She was learning for the first time in her life what it meant in feeling to begin a new phase of her life around ending another. In the final hour, she ended by taking over the curing role when she said, "Now remember, doctor, if you ever get into trouble and need any help, be sure to let me know."

Two adult dreams illustrate the same evidence of movement in the ending phase. A woman, toward the end of treatment, dreamed she went for an automobile ride accompanied by the therapist. At the top of a hill, which was reached with considerable effort, she climbed out of the machine into one that was waiting and went off, waving good-by. When she told the dream, her relaxed and smiling manner indicated she needed no one to tell her what that dream meant. Not only did she know what it meant, but she was able to act on her knowledge and set a time for her final appointment.

The other dream, again from an adult patient, also made use of an automobile. She was driving along a road by herself and had four flat tires. In the dream she was quite worried as she sat wondering what she could do. In telling the dream she said with a knowing smile, "You know what I did, in that dream? I got out and fixed the tires myself and went on my way." This woman had considerable anxiety about ending and had been questioning her ability to stand on her own feet. She answered that question to her own satisfaction in the dream.

Around the ending it is common for both adults and children to describe dreams that have in their content scenes of being born or of having a child to take care of. These dreams are closely related to the new which they feel in themselves and for which they can begin to be responsible. Just before his final appointment, a man described the following dream. In the dream he was awakened to discover someone had left a little baby boy in his room. At first it seemed very small and helpless but it changed to being much larger and older. He was baffled and wondered how he was going to take care of it but in the dream he never doubted that it was his job and that he would find a way to do it. When he told the dream to the therapist, he made his own interpretation and referred to the child as the growing sense of his own newness and added, "I am beginning to know how it feels to end."

Dreams provide an important medium of communication in therapeutic work, and this is particularly true in the ending period. The content of the dream, when understood in terms of the particular experience a child is having with the therapist, can be utilized to give both child and therapist a clearer picture of where they now are in their relationship.[7] Naturally, dreams mean more than this and many of the child's dreams seem to have little to do with the therapeutic experience. But it is significant that so many of the dreams children bring to the therapist have an important bearing on what they are doing in this particular phase of their lives. The therapist is in a strategic position to give meaning to the feeling content of these dreams around what is happening in the therapeutic relationship. He can help these children to bring the feeling out of the dream medium into the more immediate living reality of the therapeutic hour.

Considerable ending material has been discussed in other chapters, particularly in the complete cases given in the fifth

---

[7] Utilizing dream content this way in the therapeutic experience harmonizes with the way play activity is used to give meaning to the immediate experience. This use of play activity was discussed in Chapter V.

and sixth chapters. I shall now give more detail on the case whose beginning interview was discussed in Chapter IV. In this also we can see how the ending process is an integral part of the whole therapeutic process and is to be understood only as it is related to the movement throughout the case.

Bob,[8] a fearful and determined child, had moved rapidly in the first treatment hours, and his weekly appointments had become the central event in his life. The mother, who was so ready for Bob to move out of the narrow confines of his relation to her, described his eager anticipation of coming and how he retold to her the minute details of each hour.

There were several weeks in which Bob tested out the natural limits of each hour, in his struggle around time and his attempts to find out who was the boss. Against each new limit Bob vigorously asserted his own strength. It was only as he became sure of the therapist's strength that he became freer to assert and to fight. He was finding a way of being strong in relation to a person whose strength he could use and rely upon. This was a strength which did not overwhelm him but which did not melt before the force of his own efforts. He was finding a way of being a child in a relationship with an adult as an important step in discovering the values in being himself. He became very possessive and wrote a sign "keep out," openly asserting his desire "to come and live here."

Bob made interesting use of his mother to balance his relation with the therapist. If Bob made anything for the therapist he would then talk about what he had made for his mother. He had barely enough self to distribute between the mother and the therapist, and considerable guilt was stirred

[8] Bob, the second case discussed in Chapter IV, is continued here with the emphasis on the ending phase.

as his more total relationship with the mother in part broke up through the growth he could allow in his therapeutic relationship. To like two people at one time had been difficult for him. Each person he loved absorbed his total self, as he tried to live on this all-or-none principle. It was that which was beginning to break up as he found here he could have a relationship with more than one person in his life. This was growth for him.

In his ninth hour Bob said that he wanted to take the therapist home with him, but stressed the difficulties in getting to his house. "If you want to come where I am, you will have a lot of steps to climb." So his first move out of this intense relation took the therapist along with him. There was little risk in this desire as he was leaving nothing behind, but there was implicit in the assertion some ending implications which became much more definite in his next hour. It was about this time that he asserted, "If you are not here when I arrive, I will come in any way." This also carried his early feeling of being a person apart from the therapist.

His tenth hour was an important one for him. The full meaning of this hour will be clearer if we keep in mind the undifferentiated quality in this child when he started. Bob had so little awareness of being a boy; he was just a part of his mother. To be a boy would have meant the acceptance of his own difference and he fought against that. The mother fitted into this as she needed the boy almost as much as he needed her. Their lives were closely interwoven.

Bob started the hour by taking over some incompleted construction work left by another boy. He made sure it was the work of a boy and that it was all right for him to finish it. There was less need to assert his rights and more acceptance of having some rights of his own. Then he said, "This furniture is for girls and I am going to put it up for sale." Bob called out of the window: "Four cents for the whole set." "Things for girls for sale—come and get them." The differentiation between the toys for boys and those for girls carried his new feeling about himself. In this assertion of his own masculine self, Bob was giving his first open indication of being through with treatment. The comment was made: "Bob, you certainly are through with those things, maybe you are about through with this place." He was interested but puzzled and asked "why." The therapist observed, "You don't usually sell things you need," and Bob agreed to this and proceeded with the sale. He lined them along an open window sill and called to a woman who was outside: "Do you have any girls who want to buy this stuff?" Bob was not too sure of putting only girls' things up for sale and considered adding a few things for boys in the sale. He finally did not do that.

The mother's comment about him at this time was that "he seems to have gained such a possession of his masculine self." His therapeutic hour certainly showed real strides in that direction.

A new and final phase was ushered in after this interview. A plan was agreed upon that Bob would have four more appointments, and he then began to struggle against his own readiness to end. He found a new toy gun, and said: "I like to play with this and I am coming a long, long time." In addition he centered his struggle on the clock and the clock hands were pushed forward and then back. In these activities he brought out how he wanted to leave early, but at the same time he asserted his desire to stay longer than his regular time. Bob was able, however, to adhere to the decision to come "four more times." But as soon as he reaffirmed this ending plan his turmoil reappeared in another form. "I will come until I am nine." That was against his real desire because he quickly asked, "Will that be more than four Saturdays?" and was quite sarcastic when the therapist thought there would be many more Saturdays before he was that old. At the end of this strenuous but moving hour, Bob brought his mother back to see the new toy. He had never done this before because he had never been sure enough of his place in this experience to share it that openly with the mother.

After this hour, a break of two weeks was brought about by sickness and his reaction to his illness was strongly colored by the turmoil he was having around ending. Bob projected the reason for ending on the therapist, and he kept repeating to his mother, "He won't let me come more than four more times." But there was at the same time considerable comfort in finding that much strength in his therapist who could be used to carry part of the ending responsibility.

A similar ambivalence characterized his next hour. The toy continued to be useful: "When this thing goes, then I'll go." But Bob was full of his own feeling of growing and spontaneously said, "When I'm grown up, I'll be as big as my mother." Then he denied wanting to be big: "I want to stay as I am, I don't want to grow any more." But behind all these reactions he held to his decision about the final hour.

The final hour brought more pulling back and forth. In ending his therapeutic hours, Bob was ending his more infantile way of living and he seemed clearly aware of this. In action, particularly at home, he was full of the life characteristic of an eight-year-old boy but in words he still asserted, "I want to stay like Peter Pan." This came out as he was making a large pile of blocks, and with real enthusiasm spoke of it as "being the biggest thing I have ever made in my life."

In his second hour, Bob had brought a mask and had left it at the clinic. Several times he had spoken of taking it home but he was never able to do so. The mask had great meaning for him in terms of what he was and what he had become.

In the next to the last hour, he reached a decision on that mask and said: "I am never going to take that home—I'll leave it here," and he did. In leaving the mask, he was separating himself from an old quality in himself that could never face a world of people. He was now out in the open, and while there was anxiety awakened by these changes, the feeling stemmed from living more naturally. It was more the anxiety which emerges from feeling the responsibility for a new self which ending required him to assume.

Bob's final hour was quite difficult for him. Because of the break caused by his sickness there was some confusion in time. He wanted it to be his last but he tried hard to utilize the mix up to gain another hour. In every act, he seemed through with treatment. He was in and out of the room; the door was left wide open, and many references were made to the nice day outside. But he insisted: "Next week I might come if I don't have anything to do." The therapist did not allow him to end on such a vague possibility and held Bob to the earlier decision that this would be his last hour. Even though he was somewhat angry, he said "good-by" and left with his mother.

A month later he wanted to come back for one more visit and it was an easy hour with all of the struggle gone. The therapist commented: "We didn't quite get finished in that last hour, did we?" and he replied in a half-hearted manner: "I haven't finished at all." As his final act, he repeated some earlier behavior and climbed in and out of the space under the desk. Each time he called attention to the fact, "I got out myself." The therapist commented, in support of his remark, "Yes, Bob, you got in the hole and you can get out by yourself." And he replied in good masculine terms, "Darned right I can."

A year later, when he came for another visit, he used the hour to have a good time and, while a little shy in the beginning, he soon was at ease. He made no mention of wanting to come again. He really was through.

The ending is not only an affirmation of change by a child but it also involves the realization that is more difficult for some children that the change has been accelerated through the influence of the therapist. For some children, this is difficult to accept, particularly if their energies have been directed toward gaining a full sense of ownership of their own capacity to do all the changing.

John, a ten-year-old boy brought out this ending dilemma quite clearly when he said, "I sort of feel I will not give up my worries before I go away this summer, I sort of think of not giving them up, I have enough proof that what I worry about is not true. I guess you can imagine why I don't give them up." When John was encouraged to give his own reason, he said, "Because I am not quite ready to." The difficulty he was having in accepting help for his persistent and determined fears was discussed, and John then indicated he thought he would give up worrying in the summer, which he knew would be after his last interview. John had to cling to the *idea* of worrying until he was away from the therapist. Then he could feel free to show in his own everyday living the evidence that he had changed. This did not mean he was not doing a great deal in the therapeutic relationship. John had relinquished his persistent use of fear to control everyone about him and had developed a more open use of this determination in his therapeutic hour to control, by the use of a date, his final giving in to his own maturing self. John actually did more about finally giving up his worrisome behavior after he had finished. The therapist had helped him to arrive at a point where he was ready to be the different self he had achieved. The proof of this in his own living had to be under the controls he himself set. But he was through with therapy, even though he continued for a time some of the symptoms which brought him in the first place.

Children frequently wait to clear up a particular symptom after they end the actual visits with the therapist. John gave an important answer to the question as to why this happens. The disappearance or the persistence of certain symptoms cannot be used as the only guide by which the ending of treatment is determined. The real guide comes from the therapist's sensitivity about the meaning of what a child is doing in the relationship itself. The fact of his improved behavior in other aspects of his life are important when understood as a part of the child's growth with the therapist. It is true that a child's symptoms may disappear early in treatment but that is, in itself, no indication of his readiness to affirm in himself the capacities he has learned to use to effect change. A ten-year-old boy who was rebelling against school and was on the point of failing came to his second hour and announced: "There was something you said last time that made me want to do my school work. I still don't like school, but I am doing better work." He was using the therapist to explain his sudden shift, but this was merely the beginning of helping him to gain a sense of his own desire and capacity to be different. When he was really ending he announced: "I don't get along very well with girls. I don't know why. You have helped me on a lot of things, I want to figure this out for myself." So he set a task for himself and in his final hours used the improvement he described in his relation to girls as the evidence that he was now ready to accept responsibility for himself.

The discussion of this important phase of therapy will be rounded out by returning to the case of Bill whose problem and beginning reactions are discussed in Chapter V. Bill used play materials exclusively to dramatize his projections. He did it with such realism, and his phantasied characters carried so much of his feeling that the only possible relation with him was through the characters of his play. He used a steady flow of words and expressed outwardly little feeling of his own to establish his therapeutic relationship. This was particularly true throughout the first half of his therapeutic experience, and the type of interviews given in Chapter V were repeated week after week. The characters changed but the use Bill made of them to carry his own disturbed feelings was rarely altered. "Good" and "bad" were placed in constant opposition. Sometimes the good overpowered the bad, but just as frequently the bad came out on top. Nearly every hour ended with a dramatic destruction of whatever he had built during the hour.

Bill's progress toward being a better-integrated boy was indicated in the nature of his activity. In the last half of his treatment period he dropped his vivid and intensely serious phantasy play and engaged entirely in construction activity. He made boxes, book ends and calendars. While he seemed unaware of what went on about him, yet he was immediately sensitive to any change in time, any new thing another child had left behind, and at the end he recalled the exact day he had started. In each hour Bill always insisted on having his full time.

The shift from activity that was mainly destructive to a dominantly constructive interest came abruptly and it was hard to tell exactly what brought it about. But the clue may be in the vivid phantasy play in the hour just preceding the change. Bill had begun the hour drawing valentines, and placed two hearts together. He could not allow the positive implications of this drawing to stand and said: "These hearts are mad at each other." The animated phantasy that followed presented the struggle between these two hearts. One heart vigorously attacked the other and this attack, which he described with gory detail, ended this way: "The soldier [one of the hearts became a soldier] only wants to make him cry—he doesn't want to kill him." In this attack, the heart finally ran to his mother [9] and got well, and all his wounds were healed. The soldier was put in jail and the heart lived happily ever after. The heart died and went to heaven where the soldier could not hurt him.

The effort to make the heart cry seemed to have great meaning for this boy who had been so incapable of experiencing feeling in any real way. There was in him the craving to have feelings that would allow a more real relation with others. Bill's therapeutic hours were of great significance for him, but he could never share any direct expression of how he felt. All his phantasied characters were constantly invested with the most varied and intense emotional reactions that he wanted for himself.

The phantasy continued in this important hour and Bill created another soldier to attack a house with people in it. Then a train was attacked and the soldier was caught. He made a vigorous verbal attack on the bad soldier who was tortured in various ways and finally was put in the electric chair and allowed to burn. Bill gloried over the suffering as he represented it by a piece of clay placed on a hot radiator. The bad soldier was finally killed and boiled and eaten by the good soldier. This amazing hour ended with the bad soldier left in his burnt state as the good soldier went to heaven. He dramatized this by throwing a piece of clay which stuck on the ceiling.

Bill was deeply disturbed over the "bad" in himself, and, so many times in his activity, the bad, which was a projection of himself, was annihilated only to come back in a different form. He could not let the "bad" remain dead. In this hour, the cannibalistic scene which portrayed the "good" soldier

[9] Bill had been unable to express any positive feeling with his mother.

eating some of the "bad" may have meant a more natural merging of these two qualities which had been set in such vigorous opposition in himself. As long as they were maintained as such powerful and separate forces fighting each other, there could be no solution and no peace for the boy. This hour brought, for the first time, a form of activity which symbolized some incorporation of both. The "good" soldier could eat some of the "bad" in the other and still remain good.

Whether it had this meaning or not it is difficult to say with certainty. But the fact that Bill's activity changed so abruptly from this point on was clear indication that he had settled a long-standing conflict and had arrived at a more peaceful feeling in himself. Never before, in his vivid play which accurately mirrored his own inner conflict, did he allow any partial qualities in any of his characters. The all-or-none principle prevailed in his play just as it had dominated his feeling in all his everyday activities.

For three months, his weekly hours were filled with construction activity. Sometimes Bill came with an idea but more frequently the idea was provided by something he found in the office. There was one interview, however, just preceding a vacation break, which was quite different and showed how quickly he reacted to an ending he was not ready for. Bill had considerable feeling about this temporary interruption of his relationship with the therapist but could only handle the feeling in the medium of play. A porcelain baby was animated into a small baby who was to be kidnaped. The kidnapers were not going to kill the baby but were going to cover it completely in clay, leaving out only the mouth and face. Bill explained this "as more cruel than killing the baby." Again the emphasis was on trying to make the baby cry. His usual storm came up and the baby started to cry but "it is not hurt very much." The emphasis was on the cruelty of the kidnapers, who "are not going to feed the baby but she is not going to die." They torture the baby by hanging her upside down saying, "You know babies don't like to be upside down but they want to do the cruelest things."

It was quite clear that all this feeling was roused by the temporary ending. Bill was not ready and knew it in his own feeling, and the drama of the hour showed this. To be left at this point was the cruel act, and it seemed to him as if he were being smothered. The therapist's going away was a virtual stealing of his precious time. But Bill made it clear that the baby did not die, even though cruelly treated.

The therapist attempted to bring this feeling into the immediate reality and commented about Bill's disturbance over being left. Bill stopped his play, looked at the therapist with his tense and serious expression, said nothing and went on with a different set of characters. This was about as close as he could get to any actual expression of the feeling that arose. There was a lighter tone to the latter part of the hour as he substituted a sausage for the baby. Bill actually laughed and got some fun out of this play.

The last hour before the break brought a return of the construction work, and Bill made a little box saying, "It is going to be a little box to keep things in." He took the box with him.

Following the summer break there were thirteen more interviews with Bill. He quickly settled down to making things and gave minute descriptions of each step. He rarely asked for any help, but always was acutely aware of the therapist's presence. Rarely was Bill at a loss for something to do and in one hour, when he had become less interested in what he was doing, the subject of ending came up for discussion. The therapist had to initiate the subject as Bill was too absorbed in what he was doing to be aware of the actual meaning of his growing in terms of ending. This had to be initiated in order to help Bill experience more of the feeling he was not ready to express openly. His better adjustment to his life in his school and to his group and the moderately successful visits to his home, which was in another city, indicated his need and readiness to affirm his change through ending this therapeutic relationship.

Bill was disturbed by the discussion and first said, "I want to come in for a few years yet," adding, "My mother wants me to come." This was one of the rare times he had mentioned his parents. Two interviews later, he was able to take part in deciding on a date, and chose his birthday, saying, "I came back on my birthday." He referred here to his return after the first long break and he was correct. This gave him seven more interviews.

There was little change in his activity until the next to his last hour when Bill volunteered a comment that the next time was to be his last, and added, "I think I will come in again sometime, maybe in one or two years." Then he wanted to know how long he had been coming and remembered his first visit saying, "The reason I came was I could not get along very well with the kids; now I can." This was the first time this boy had made any direct reference to his difficulties at home and at school. It was also the first open recognition of his own change.

Bill gave the same recognition of his change in his therapeutic hours by describing the shift in his activity, and of this he volunteered: "At first, I built farms on the floor and had babies in the houses; now I make things with wood and paint posters."

His last hour [10] was most unusual and significant because

---

[10] Brief reference was made to this final hour in the author's article "Participation in Therapy," published as part of a symposium on "Trends in Therapy," *Journal of Orthopsychiatry*, v. IX no. 4 (October, 1939), p. 742.

he condensed into it so much of what he had done over a long period of therapy. He started by asking: "Do you remember the date when I came the first time?" The therapist found this for him. Then he asked: "Did you find out what I did the first time I came?" and it seemed so important for Bill to know the detail that the therapist fitted into the unusualness of the hour and brought out the record. He had always been aware of the therapist's note-taking which, in this case, did not interfere with his relationship to the boy. Together, they went over the details recorded in the record and Bill added more about the zoo, the bad elephant, the bad hunter, the farm and the baby. Words are inadequate to describe the feeling this boy had as he went over the detail of one hour after another.

When Bill had spent half of his hour in this, he said: "You know what I will do today? I think I will go back to the old time and make things with clay. I am going to make an old house, make a baby, and there is going to be a toilet. It will be an old house just like the one I made a long time ago." In recapturing the old feeling about himself, he was quite aware of the new quality he now had found.

He duplicated all the detail of the first hour that had happened two years earlier but there was a very different feeling quality in it. Now he was really related to the therapist with a more mature feeling about himself. But the content and words were the same. The house was old, the roof leaked and, "the poor baby is going to cry." He made it clear "they are not bad people, they are just poor."

The scene changed with the passage of two months. Again it was stormy and hail came down and hit the baby and she began to cry. The roof began to fall and the mother grabbed the baby, covered it up, and then the house fell down. Next they were outside and had no house. The feeling content of this seemed closely related to Bill's ending and being left out in the cold. The father was dead but just as the house fell down a rich man came along. "He is not a robber, he is a good man." He took them to his house where there is no "rotten lumber."

But as he was taking them away, the bad robber appeared. He had a gun and started to shoot. "But the rich man is strong and grabs the gun away from the robber, kills the robber and then they lived happily. They are just as happy now as they were when the father was living. Now the robber is killed, the rich man can throw the gun away because he would not need it any more." A moment later he said good-by and his therapeutic experience was over.

In ending this meaningful relationship, he dramatized the greater sense of unity in himself. He portrayed the baby as grown-up and as having found his place in relationships with others. This represented Bill's feeling about himself, and the long-standing dilemma created by his good and bad split had a more settled solution. With this new feeling, he was able to end this unique experience in which he had found himself.

Four years later, while attending a boarding school for normal boys he wrote to his therapist and said in part: "My favorite study is biology. It is extremely interesting for we learn about the lives and reproduction of all kinds of animals. We have studied amoebae, algae, flowers and lots of other things. The meals are swell and it is time to eat so I will close." It was a very natural letter of a thirteen-year-old boy.

Children use the therapeutic experience to relive past periods of their development which failed to give the satisfaction necessary to enable them to move on to more mature periods. One child may have to be the infant again in this experience before he can go on to a more creative use of the more mature self which a therapist can help him find. The therapist can help him do that if he is firmly oriented to the growth-inducing values of the immediate experience. Then he can start where the child is, in feeling, and assist him to grow from that point. The ending of therapy then can be what it should be, the affirmation of a more responsible feeling about the self, gained in the differentiating steps of the relationship which the therapist has enabled the child to establish.

Without doubt the neurotic boy just described had indulged in these same phantasies in the isolation of his playroom. But for him there was no growth in such activity. He could bring all these phantasies into connection with a living reality in his therapeutic hours, and the therapy was in this and not in the particular content of each hour.

In bringing this chapter to a close, an essential point, made many times throughout the material in one way or another, needs to be repeated. The child or adolescent, or even the adult, can infantilize this new relationship if that is his need. He can grow from that base and use the therapist as a symbol of a new reality in the present world in which the patient is trying to acquire a more grown-up feeling in keeping with his real status. But when the therapist infantilizes this experience by holding the focus on the past, he confuses the unique and strategic influence he can represent to a patient who is trying to use him to become free of the past. Therapy is an awakening process, but if the waking up is not in the world of immediate reality of people and events, it is not a waking up but a new medium to continue a dream existence.

10

BROADER IMPLICATIONS OF A
THERAPEUTIC PHILOSOPHY

CHILDREN CAN be helped to help themselves. Like the opening theme of a symphony which is given varied treatment through its several movements, the philosophy of therapy that has been developed throughout the material of this book returns in a final summing up to emphasize some of the broader implications of therapy.

The life process exists only in and through the individual. This truth is often submerged or pushed aside in modern complicated social structures where the place of the individual is undergoing cataclysmic modification. Throughout the world, the place and value of the individual are in jeopardy. It is equally true that the therapeutic process, as a segment of the larger living reality, occurs only in and through the individual who, by his participation, enables therapy to happen. The life process leads to the emergence of individual differences, and the therapeutic process is an episode in life experience, the goal of which is to help the individual to be himself [1] in a world of other and different human beings. Just as there can be no life apart from life, there can be no conception of therapy that is not closely

---

[1] Throughout this book I have stressed that this is possible only as the individual feels and values his relatedness to others. Being an individual carries a responsibility to the group as well as to the self.

interwoven in the life experiences of the individual concerned.

The principles of therapy are not altogether new. Each generation not only creates the new but deepens and enriches the meaning of the old. Theories and interpretations may change but there is a core of continuity to human experience that remains the same. Therapy as a technical development belongs to our present century but the understanding of the implications of therapy, conceived as it is in this book as a growth experience, is not alone of this generation. Plato's *Republic* written twenty-three hundred years ago developed, in the allegory of the cave, an understanding of human psychological growth which seems to me to throw light on the therapeutic process of the present day.[2]

In the following dialogue the natural condition of man so far as education and ignorance are concerned is compared to a state of things like the following: "Imagine a number of men living in an underground cavernous chamber with an entrance open to the light extending along the entire length of the cavern in which they have been confined from their childhood, with their legs and necks so shackled that they are obliged to sit still and forward—and imagine a bright fire burning way off, above and behind them, and an elevated roadway passing between the fire and the prisoners, with a low wall along it, like the screens which conjurers put up in front of their audience and above which they exhibit their wonders."

"I have it," he replied.

"Also figure to yourself a number of persons walking behind this wall and carrying with them statues of men and images of other animals—together with various other articles

[2] *The Republic of Plato*, translated into English by John Dewelyn Davies and David James Vaughan, Book VII (Macmillan & Co., Ltd., London, 1925), pp. 235-7.

which overtop the wall, and let some of the passers-by be talking and others silent."

"You are describing a strange scene and strange prisoners."

"They resemble us," I replied. "For let me ask you in the first place whether persons so confined could have seen anything of themselves or of each other beyond the shadows thrown by the fire upon the cavern facing them."

"Certainly not."

"And is not their knowledge of the things carried past them equally limited? And if they were able to converse with one another do you not think that they would be in the habit of giving names to the objects which they saw before them?"

"Doubtless they would."

"And if their prison house returned an echo whenever one of the passers-by opened his lips, to what could they refer the voice if not to the shadow which was passing."

"Unquestionably they would refer it to that."

"Then surely such persons would hold the shadows of the manufactured articles to be the only realities."

"Without a doubt they would."

"Now consider what would happen if the course of nature brought them release from their fetters in the following manner. Suppose one of them has been released and compelled suddenly to stand up and turn his neck around and walk with open eyes toward the light, and let us suppose he goes through all these actions with pain and that the dazzling splendor renders him incapable of discerning those objects of which he used formerly to see the shadows. What answer should you expect him to make if someone were to tell him that in those days he was watching foolish phantoms but that now he is somewhat nearer to reality and is turned toward things more real and sees more correctly . . . should you not expect him to be puzzled and regard his old visions as truer than the objects now forced upon his notice?"

"Yes, much truer."

"And if he were further compelled to gaze at the light itself, would not his eyes be distressed and would he not shrink and turn away to the things which he could see distinctly and consider them to be really clearer than the things pointed to him?"

"Just so."

"And if someone were to drag him violently up the tough and steep ascent from the cavern and refuse to let him go back till he had drawn him out into the light of the sun would he not, think you, be vexed and indignant at such treatment and on reaching the light would he not find his eyes so dazzled by the glare as to be incapable of making out so much as one of the objects that are now called true?"

"Yes, he would find it so at first."

"Hence, I suppose, habit will be necessary to enable him to perceive objects in the upper world. At first he must be successful in distinguishing shadows; then he will discern the reflections of men and other things in water, and afterward the realities; and after this he will raise his eyes to encounter the light of the moon and the stars finding it less difficult to study the heavenly bodies and the heaven itself by night, than the sun and sun's light by day. Last of all I imagine he will be able to observe and contemplate the nature of the sun, not as it appears in *water*, but as it *is* in itself in its own territory."

While, as I have said, psychological therapy is of our day, the principles of therapy cannot be altogether new since they are rooted in what is essential in all living and learning. Plato had a sounder understanding of this. In this dialogue he presented not only the nature of the life situations needing change but the nature of the experience necessary if the individual is to find in himself the new realities symbolized by the therapist who, to a troubled child or adult, represents the present world of reality. The individual is forced by various motivations to take the first steps out of the cavern of the past. With a child the parent may activate the forces that pull him to his feet and usually it is the parent who accompanies him in his first steps toward the dazzling light of a new reality. The parent will be motivated in this direction by the variety of influences impinging upon him and crystallized in the first stages of the clinical journey. The new for which he reaches out may be illuminated with a light that is too dazzling and may bring temporary retreat into the cavern from which he is trying to escape. The child may be dragged up the steps in a manner that Plato describes. Certainly the new into which he emerges will be at first discerned through values and terms that describe the only reality he knows; necessarily he will be vexed and fearful, particularly if the efforts are directed toward making him describe the new in terms familiar to the person to whom he is exposed but strange to him who has only known the shadows of a past he has been unable to relinquish.

The therapist symbolizes the new into which the individual emerges either through the inexorable demands of his own basic desires or through the demands of the culture whose shadows move before him. It is the therapist who stands for a strength in the individual, the values of which he has not fully experienced in a reality that both allows and requires their creative use. In him are represented the light and meaning of the present, and freedom from the shackles that bind individuals to a past which has no life of its own, but only shadows and phantasies whose reality depends on darkness. Many human beings never emerge from the cavernous depths of this devitalized past. Others make a move to emerge but retreat in fear or resentment.

For many individuals of our day, the therapist has come to symbolize the forces of life which they both want and fear. Such a therapist needs the wisdom of Plato to know that while the child or adult patient is emerging from the neurotic unreality of the past he could neither use nor go beyond, that at first he will describe the new to which he is now exposed in terms of the shadows which to him still have more reality. But the therapist can never forget that he is not sitting on the seat in the cavern with the child. The therapist remains the symbol of the new even though the child's discernment of him is couched in terms of another reality. Forgetting this tends to destroy the therapeutic influence by drawing the therapist back into the "cavern" with the child. As a therapist he stands out in the brilliant light of a present into which the child has emerged, or to which he has been impelled.

When the therapist himself is oriented to the realities of the illuminated world of the present, he can allow and encourage the child to discern him through the realities of the child's own experience. The therapist may be seen by the child as the shadow without becoming the shadow. The child may attempt to maintain his place on the seat in the cavern by drawing the therapist back with him. The child may be unable to leave the fettered world, or may seek return to the familiar and lifeless realm of the cavern. But, as I have said, the therapist cannot help the child by going back with him. He can help the child only as long as he can maintain his place as a living symbol of the world of action and feeling. Then the help can be directed toward the emerging strength of the child who first discerns the shadows of the old and then the images of the new and finally "as himself in his own territory." The differentiation inherent in a therapeutic growth experience has been achieved when he has found that place which is his; then the course of his own development can proceed without the therapist who no longer is a symbol but a reality whose help is no longer needed.

A therapeutic philosophy that stems from a belief in the creativeness of human difference has implications that extend far beyond the specific area of childhood. Therapy with children is concerned with an experience in which the child gains a more valid feeling for the self he has and which he can relate, with growing satisfaction, to the day-by-day relationships within his family and community. The successful outcome of a therapeutic experience for a child is one in which he has found that he can be the child he is in a relationship with an adult. The dignity of his own littleness can be expressed and felt around the bigness of the adult which can be used to define and give meaning to the child's feeling of difference. The world of the child and the world of the adult become interwoven each with its own value because they are arrived at together. Thomas Mann [8] seems to say this same thing in the following passage: "But lo, the world hath many centres, one for each created being, and about each one it lieth in its own circle. Thou standest but half an ell from me, yet about thee lieth a universe whose centre I am not but thou art. Therefore both are true, according as one speaketh from thy centre or from mine. And I, on the other hand, stand in the centre of mine. For our universes are not far from each other so that they do not touch; rather hath God pushed them and interwoven them deep into each other, so that you Ishmaelites *do indeed journey quite independently and according to your own ends, whither you will, but besides that you are the means and tool, in our interwovenness, that I arrive at my goal.*" (Italics mine.)

Essential differences in adult and child can never be defined or experienced in isolation. The very nature of living

[8] Mann, Thomas, *Joseph in Egypt* (New York, Alfred Knopf, 1938), v. I, p. 4.

does not allow this, since life has no meaning except as it is in relation to life and a setting. Differences are broadly defined for an infant before experience. He is born into a preformed culture and the character of his early life has this "given" quality, irrespective of desire. His responses to these realities, however, provide the important dynamic quality to his growth. The child begins to achieve for himself a feeling for his place in the world to which he belongs. The child's own participation makes these realities of mother and father and surroundings a part of the self he begins to feel as his own. The life of another continues in him in some measure, but in continuing there appears a new emergent in the self of the child. He will be more than the sum of all that goes before, as the whole is always different from the sum of its parts. He will be more than a recapitulation of the thousands of years that have preceded him, and far more than mere imitator and repeater of the lives of his parents. He has the capacity to become different from anything that has preceded him, and in his growth he can and must acquire some sense of his own responsibility to determine the direction of his destiny. I realize this is seriously questioned today in a world in which the individual seems so tossed about by forces in which he has no part, that seem and are the denial of the fundamental respect for the individual from which democracy stems. But I feel strongly that it is more important today than ever before to affirm with the clarity of clinical support, a belief in the individual's capacity to be responsible for his own direction within the structure of the culture in which he lives.

The therapeutic experience is an episode in the journey of some children toward the realization of the potentialities that lie within themselves. It is a temporary expression of living made necessary by the variety of reactions that reveal stopovers on the journey toward self-fulfillment. The therapist becomes the prototype of the continuum in development, a symbol of an opportunity to resume the journey once again —a journey that can be taken only with the participation of the traveler who needs stimulus to leave the sidetrack and turn his vision ahead toward the new and unknown and away from the old in which he has been waylaid or where he has overstayed his time. The urge to grow that is universal in all living matter provides motivation for the journey. The therapist never actually supplies this but he is part of the coming to life of this energy which the individual has within himself but which he has been, until now, unable to use effectively. In the journey the child may want to make the therapist the engine that does all the work. He may try to pull back, or to reverse his own direction. These variations of the new movement with many children gradually are worked out to the point where the child can leave the therapist to continue his journey among those who naturally belong to the party with whom he travels.

The therapeutic experience must not be mistaken for the journey itself, although it may be one important phase of it. But it is only a part, and has worth because it is integrated into concurrent aspects of the child's growth. When this journey is taken off into the hills or down in the caverns of the past, and as a side trip quite unrelated to the realities that exist simultaneously, its meaning as a growth-inducing experience will fail. It is the interwovenness that is so essential for the child and parent who have lost their bearings and have sought the service of a pilot to get back on the main course to which they themselves can then adhere when the pilot has finally fulfilled his function.

As I have said previously, we are going through a period in history when the status of the individual is undergoing great change. In large sections of the world he has ceased to have value except as he contributes to mass security. To become different, which is the inherent direction of all human development, threatens this pseudohomogeneity which can only be developed by a suppression of difference. The child under such totalitarian conceptions is fashioned as a tool of the state, and the family, as the "cultural workshop," has its functions pre-empted, with loyalties turned toward the impersonal state with its idealized leader.

Totalitarian philosophy stems not only from insecurity in human beings, but even more from the exploitation of natural insecurities found in all people. The greater the uncertainties in life, the more will individuals seek their source of safety in the organized state that exists for their welfare. A state that seeks to perpetuate itself by the exploitation of human weakness will seek to build a conception of the mass or racial self that must be preserved from the "aggressions" of those who are different. Differences cannot be tolerated in individuals, as they become a threat to homogeneity which must be achieved if mass strength is to be sustained. The vicious cycle of such a philosophy becomes apparent. It leads, in turn, to greater weaknesses requiring still more protection from the state and greater intolerance of all divergent elements that threaten from without.

The oft-quoted slogan, "In unity there is strength" holds but a half-truth. If unity is achieved only by the destruction of individual strengths that go to make up a social order, then the false unity becomes itself a new source of weakness. Real unity, whether in the family or in larger national groups, can only emerge as individuals find creative worth in their own differences, which thus enable them "to live and let live." A child in a family becomes a source of potential strength when he is helped to be a person in his own right. Then, and only then, can he become responsible for the direction and use of the energy which he has, and contribute to the social order in which he moves and has his being.

There is great need in the world today for a philosophy, whether therapeutic or more broadly social, that stems from a recognition and acceptance of individual difference. The therapeutic point of view, of which I have written, in this book has its roots deep in a concept of individual responsibility. Its recurrent theme is that individuals can be helped to help themselves. At a time when the world needs new orientation to the essential place of the individual, we need to emphasize the strengths of human nature and its capacity for self-responsibility. This is implicit in a therapeutic philosophy which is built around the strengths and spontaneities which the individuals, both child and adult, have for effecting changes and for assuming responsibility for their own individual differences and development. It would be truistic, or meaningless, if it could not be translated into clinical procedures that allow the therapist to assist the child or adult coming for help to gain a sense of his individual worth and integrity. When psychotherapy becomes, thus, a living experience, it has implications far broader than the results achieved in individual cases.

I have attempted, from first to last in the material of this book, to emphasize in various ways this essential theme: a child can be helped to help himself. Only through his own participation can the changes that have been effected have meaning that can be interwoven into the fabric of his day-to-day living. When the child has been helped to affirm the value of what he is in an active, changing world, his major focus of interest has been directed ahead and away from the shackles of an outlived past. There is implicit in this an affirmation of a philosophy of responsibility, and a belief in the dignity of human nature as it exists.

INDEX